Nightingale's Vision: Advancing the Nursing Profession Beyond 2020

by Sue Johnson, PhD, RN, NE-BC

American Nurses Association
Silver Spring, Maryland • 2017

The America Nurses Association (ANA) is the premier organization representing the interests of the nation's 3.6 million registered nurses. ANA advances the nursing profession by fostering high standards of nursing practice, promoting a safe and ethical work environment, bolstering the health and wellness of nurses, and advocating on health care issues that affect nurses and the public. ANA is at the forefront of improving the quality of health care for all.

American Nurses Association
8515 Georgia Avenue, Suite 400
Silver Spring, MD 20910-3492
1-800-274-4ANA
http://www.Nursingworld.org

Library of Congress Cataloging-in-Publication Data available on request.

978-1-935213-98-7   Print   SAN: 851-3481   05/2017
978-1-935213-99-4   ePDF
978-0-9726088-0-0   EPUB
978-0-9726088-1-7   Kindle

First printing: May 2017

Contents

Contents

Dedication

This book is dedicated to every nurse whose time and talents have and will positively impact patient-focused care. My thanks to multiple organizations and colleagues who helped the survey process succeed and every nurse and interprofessional collaborator who have informed my practice over many years. Most of all, the book is a tribute to a visionary who changed the world in health care and nursing: Florence Nightingale.

Sue Johnson, PhD, RN, NE-BC

Introduction

"A profession, a trade, a necessary occupation, something to fill and employ all my faculties, I have always felt essential to, I have always longed for, consciously or not. The first thought I can remember, and the last, was nursing work."

—F. Nightingale
(Cook, 1913a, p. 106)

Florence Nightingale established a deep and diverse foundation for professional nursing practice. Within and from that foundation have rooted and grown several generations of nursing practice, theory, and policy that continue to this day.

However robust and productive this ongoing growth, nurses can still find it helpful/useful to acknowledge it as more than simply our inheritance, our historical legacy. Nightingale's vision continues today as nursing moves into uncharted territory in a dynamic and, at times, dysfunctional, health care environment.

Today's nurse leaders must advance the profession by leveraging our past and present into a future in which nursing is a dynamic force in health care locally, regionally, nationally, and globally. The 2010 Institute of Medicine (IOM) report and the 2015 assessment of its first five years of implementation set several goals for 2020, a year that will mark the 200th birthday of the profession's founder, Florence Nightingale.

Nightingale's accomplishments that reflect the IOM recommendations:

1. Transformed nursing education by founding the first English training school at St. Thomas' Hospital in London

2. Leveraged nursing leadership by training, recommending placement, and mentoring nurse superintendents at major hospitals in England and throughout the world

3. Fostered collaboration between nurses and physicians

4. Utilized data collection and statistics to improve health care across the British Commonwealth

5. Insisted that "Nightingale Nurses" learn something every day to make progress in their careers by promoting lifelong learning

6. Emphasized that nursing practice must focus on the patient and his or her needs in care delivery redesign

The issues have changed, and nurse leaders must change their approaches and think out of the box to advance the profession beyond 2020 into a future that was undreamt of a generation ago. Yet to be addressed: How nurse leaders from 25 to 45 years of age perceive their role in nursing beyond 2020. This book now looks into this in detail in the context of the 2010 Institute of Medicine (IOM) recommendations from *The Future of Nursing* for nursing and the 2015 follow-up Assessment Report.

Beginning with Chapter 2, each chapter follows this outline to assist the reader in following Nightingale's Vision, the progress of the IOM recommendations, and the perspectives of practicing nurses from age 25 to 45.

- **Nightingale's Vision:** Following a quote by Nightingale, this section depicts a situation from her life that parallels the Institute of Medicine (IOM) recommendation described in the chapter.

- **IOM's Vision:** This section describes one of the eight 2010 IOM recommendations and plans by the IOM committee to achieve this goal (IOM, 2011).

- **Progress toward IOM's Vision:** This section addresses review findings of the 2015 Committee for Assessing Progress on Implementing the Recommendations of the IOM Report (the Study Committee). Subtopics include the following:
  - **Accomplishments:** Delineates the achievements by the Future of Nursing: Campaign for Action (the Campaign) and its 51 state Action Coalitions (National Academies of Sciences, Engineering, and Medicine, 2016, Preface ix) in the first five years (2010–2015).
  - **Challenges:** Outlines areas for improvement to achieve IOM goals.
  - **Study Committee's Conclusion:** A statement about findings related to the IOM recommendation.
  - **Study Committee's Recommendation:** A statement from the Study Committee about how to make future progress toward the IOM recommendation.

- **Nurses' Vision** [select survey questions]:
  A 15-question survey—integrating Nightingale's vision
  for the profession, the 2010 Institute of Medicine
  (IOM) recommendations for nursing and the 2015
  Assessment Report about education, nursing leadership, interprofessional collaboration, data collection/
  utilization, lifelong learning, and involvement in
  care delivery redesign—was developed via Survey
  Monkey (Appendix A). The survey was posted on
  Facebook, and a link was sent to 1,000 registered
  nurses between ages 25 and 45 throughout the
  United States in January 2017 to determine their
  knowledge of the IOM recommendations and their
  views about the future of nursing. This age group
  was selected because they will be leaders of the
  nursing profession in the 2020s and beyond. Their
  feedback will be included in each chapter and is vital
  in assessing their knowledge and perception of the
  IOM recommendations in shaping the future course
  of nursing in the United States. Two hundred and
  thirty responses were received—a 23% return—from
  34 states and the District of Columbia. To preserve
  anonymity, each response was only evaluated by
  location. Graphic depiction of response summaries
  is found in Appendix B. Each chapter describes these
  nurses' responses about the subject of that chapter.
  All comments are quoted as stated by respondents
  without commentary or judgment. Their ratings and
  insights deserve the reader's attention even in cases of
  disagreement.

Careful review of the status of each of the IOM recommendations using this framework may help nurses
develop a plan for action to advance the profession
beyond 2020. Florence Nightingale would applaud their
accomplishments.

These nursing leaders in multiple settings and in this age cohort will determine nursing's future; they must play a significant role in practice issues and the growth of the profession. Their voices must be heard and heeded for nursing to achieve Nightingale's vision for the profession and the outcomes of the IOM recommendations. This is their opportunity to be heard.

CHAPTER 1

How It Began: The Institute of Medicine (IOM) and Nursing

"God meant me for a reformer and I have turned out a detective. I have never been used to influence people except by leading in *work*; and to have to influence them by talking and writing is hard."

—F. Nightingale (Cook, 1913a, p. 251)

The National Academy of Sciences was chartered by the U.S. Congress in 1863 as a private, nonprofit group of scholars to advance science and technology for the general welfare of citizens. In 1970, the Academy created the Institute of Medicine* (IOM), where members of health

---

* The Institute of Medicine was renamed the Health and Medicine Division (HMD) of the National Academies of Sciences, Engineering, and Medicine on March 15, 2016, to continue its work in medicine and emphasize its wider focus on a range of health issues (National Academies of Science, Engineering, and Medicine, 2016).

professions examine public health policy issues; advise the government; and identify medical care, research, and education issues (IOM, 2010, p. 5). After the 2008 election, the Robert Wood Johnson Foundation (RWJF) partnered with the IOM to recommend changes in nursing education and practice to meet the demands of health system reforms. They held three information-gathering forums between 2009 and 2010 that explored nursing in acute care, in the community, and in education (IOM, 2010, p. 1). The final forum occurred one month prior to March 23, 2010, when President Barack Obama signed the law creating the Patient Protection and Affordable Care Act (IOM, 2010, Preface ix). The RWJF and the IOM realized that high-quality, accessible health care in a climate of health care reforms required outstanding care and leadership by the nation's largest health care profession: nurses.

The IOM expert panel, supplemented by RWJF staff experts in nursing, research, and communications, combined best practices and innovative approaches in the "RWJF Initiative on the Future of Nursing at the IOM" (IOM, 2011, Foreword, ix).

In late 2010, their alliance created and published a seminal work: *The Future of Nursing: Leading Change, Advancing Health* (IOM, 2011). Their recommendations included the following:

1. Remove scope-of-practice barriers (IOM, 2011, p. 9)

2. Expand opportunities for nurses to lead and diffuse collaborative improvement efforts (IOM, 2011, p. 11)

3. Implement nurse residency programs (IOM, 2011, p. 11)

4. Increase the proportion of nurses with a baccalaureate degree to 80% by 2020 (IOM, 2011, p. 12)

5. Double the number of nurses with a doctorate by 2020 (IOM, 2011, p. 13)

6. Ensure that nurses engage in lifelong learning (IOM, 2011, p. 13)

7. Prepare and enable nurses to lead change to advance health (IOM, 2011, p. 14)

8. Build an infrastructure for the collection and analysis of interprofessional health care workforce data (IOM, 2011, p. 14)

After the report and its recommendations were released, RWJF and AARP initiated a campaign—the Future of Nursing Campaign for Action—to implement these recommendations via the Center to Champion Nursing in America (CCNA). The CCNA collaborates with state Action Coalitions to meet its goals (National Academies of Sciences, Engineering, and Medicine, 2016, p. 2). The Campaign focuses on six major pillars:

1. Advancing education transformation

2. Leveraging nursing leadership

3. Removing barriers to practice and care

4. Fostering interprofessional collaboration

5. Promoting diversity

6. Bolstering workforce data (National Academies of Sciences, Engineering, and Medicine, 2016, p. 2)

In 2015, RWJF asked the IOM to evaluate progress in implementing the original eight recommendations and to recognize areas for improvement to achieve the recommendations. A new Study Committee of experts conducted an independent review of activities and results in the preceding five years. This review resulted in further delineation of the original recommendations and ideas for attainment. These additional statements included the following:

1. Build common ground around scope of practice and other issues in policy and practice (National Academies of Sciences, Engineering, and Medicine, 2016, p. 5)

2. Continue pathways toward increasing the percentage of nurses with a baccalaureate degree (National Academies of Sciences, Engineering, and Medicine, 2016, p. 8)

3. Create and fund transition-to-practice residency programs (National Academies of Sciences, Engineering, and Medicine, 2016, p. 8)

4. Promote nurses' pursuit of doctoral degrees (National Academies of Sciences, Engineering, and Medicine, 2016, p. 8)

5. Promote nurses' interprofessional and lifelong learning (National Academies of Sciences, Engineering, and Medicine, 2016, p. 9)

6. Make diversity in the nursing workforce a priority (National Academies of Sciences, Engineering, and Medicine, 2016, p. 10)

7. Expand efforts and opportunities for interprofessional collaboration and leadership development for nurses (National Academies of Sciences, Engineering, and Medicine, 2016, p. 12)

8. Promote the involvement of nurses in the redesign of care delivery and payment systems (National Academies of Sciences, Engineering, and Medicine, 2016, p. 13)

9. Communicate with a wider and more diverse audience to gain support for campaign objectives (National Academies of Sciences, Engineering, and Medicine, 2016, p. 13)

10. Improve workforce data collection (National Academies of Sciences, Engineering, and Medicine, 2016, p. 14)

Two blue ribbon expert panels have developed and refined these recommendations for nurses to impact health care in 2020 beyond Nightingale's vision and their current accomplishments. The following chapters examine the thoughts and perceptions of today's nurse leaders from 25 to 45 years of age in multiple settings and roles about the IOM recommendations and practice issues facing them as they look forward to the 2020s. Nightingale's vision will serve as a guide, and these nurses will lead us into that future era.

CHAPTER 2

Remove Scope-of-Practice Barriers (2010)

"Every brick is of consequence, every dab of mortar, that it may be as good as possible in building up your house. A chain is no stronger than its weakest link: therefore every link is of consequence. And there can be no 'small' thing in Nursing."

–F. Nightingale
(Nightingale, 2012, p. 95)

NIGHTINGALE'S VISION

Nightingale's vision of care provided by trained nurses began with her founding of the Nightingale School at St. Thomas' Hospital and continued with the establishment of additional nurse training schools. There was general agreement that nurse graduates must maintain competence to practice safely. The barrier encountered was disagreement about how this competency should be demonstrated. Some English nurses formed the British Nurses Association in 1887 and pushed for nurses' registration. Their plan was for a board to establish nurses' competence and certify their proficiency by including their names in a Register of Nurses. The board recommended that three years of training in a hospital was appropriate for this designation. Nightingale's vision of nurses' competence to perform the scope of their duties was diametrically opposed to a nurse registry. The proposal would mean that the nurse was deemed competent when her name was included. Nightingale believed that the Register reflected a minimum standard, and that was not good enough for nursing practice. She expressed concern that the decision makers for the Register had not been validated and that inclusion or exclusion might be arbitrary. She also believed that character was as vital to a nurse as technical skills. Her argument against registration reflected her belief that lifelong learning was essential for nursing competence. Her resistance stalled nurses' registration, but she was prophetic when she said, "Forty years hence, such a scheme might not be preposterous, *provided* the intermediate time be diligently and successfully employed in levelling up, that is, making all nurses at least equal to the best trained nurses of this day, and in levelling up Training Schools in like manner" (Cook, 1913b, p. 364).

IOM'S VISION

"Nurses should practice to the full extent of their education and training" (Institute of Medicine [IOM], 2011, p. 85).

The "Committee on the Robert Wood Johnson Foundation Initiative on the Future of Nursing at the Institute of Medicine" (IOM, 2011, p. 2) created a vision where achievement of truly patient-centered care required greater involvement of nurses, especially advanced practice registered nurses (APRNs). Passage of the Affordable Care Act* (ACA) in 2010 increased emphasis on wellness and prevention activities, care for patients with chronic or preexisting conditions, improved access to care by underserved populations, and averting harmful outcomes from hospital-acquired infections and preventable readmissions (IOM, 2011). The Committee believed that nurses, particularly APRNs, could

---

* As this is being written, the continued status of the ACA legislation is in doubt as Congress pursues repeal and replacement legislation.

positively impact each of these situations, resulting in more patient-focused care (IOM, 2011).

However, successful transition of nurses to an advanced leadership role in patient care required that they legally be permitted to discharge the responsibilities based on their education and reflected in their competencies and skill sets. The number of primary care physicians was decreasing and collaborative full partnerships between these physicians and APRNs were limited. Major concerns included regulatory restrictions limiting registered nurses' practice, professional opposition, health care system fragmentation, and obsolete insurance company policies (IOM, 2011).

In the United States, the practice of all health professions is regulated by state statutes and rules. Physician practice was the first health profession to have its scope of practice defined by legislation. Defined activities and responsibilities included "provisions making it illegal for anyone not licensed as a physician to undertake any of the acts included in this definition" (IOM, 2011, p. 96). Subsequently, physicians were authorized "to control the activities of other health care providers" (IOM, 2011, p. 97).

On the other hand, the scope of practice for registered nurses, including APRNs, was restricted based on each state's nurse practice act. As nurses' education grew in primary and specialty care, these regulations did not change with their increased knowledge and skills. At the time of the Committee's work, there were only "16 states plus the District of Columbia" (IOM, 2011, p. 98) in which nurse practitioners (NPs) could practice to the limits of their licenses and education without requirement of physician supervision or collaboration. NPs in these states performed primary care independently, only referring patients requiring care beyond their scope of knowledge, skills, and competencies. Other states restricted APRN practice by requiring physician oversight and written collaboration agreements as well as, in some cases, specifications for chart reviews.

Changing state nurse practice acts was an arduous process and greatly limited patients' access to care by APRN providers (IOM, 2011).

Another barrier to APRN expanded practice was the opposition voiced by the American Medical Association (AMA) nationally. The AMA opposed legislative changes in state nurse practice acts because they considered independent practice by nurses as practicing medicine without a medical license. The American Association of Family Physicians (AAFP) and other medical groups joined this opposition. The AAFP supported collaborative teams of physicians and nurses but insisted that APRNs not independently replace physicians in primary care settings.

These physician groups have cited patient safety concerns, particularly related to prescriptive authority. However, evidence has shown that APRNs are proficient in delivering effective, safe patient care and correctly and accurately prescribing medications (IOM, 2011).

Disparities in the health care system create barriers for patients seeking providers for chronic conditions and reimbursement difficulties for APRNs providing their care. When independent practice is not legally feasible, the APRN may be salaried with payment going to the physician via a collaboration agreement. Although APRNs can directly bill Medicare and Medicaid for some services, insurance companies have been reluctant to recognize them as providers for reimbursement of services. This barrier is especially onerous for nurses managing health clinics for at risk populations (IOM, 2011).

These were the issues related to registered nurses' scope of practice in 2010 when the Committee developed its recommendations. Supporting recommendations included the following:

1. Expansion of the Medicare program by Congress to include "coverage of advanced practice registered nurse

services that are within the scope of practice under applicable state law" (IOM, 2011, p. 9)

2. "Amend the Medicare program to authorize advanced practice registered nurses to" certify for home health services and admit "to hospice and skilled nursing facilities" (IOM, 2011, p. 10).

3. Revision of scope-of-practice regulations by state legislatures and requirements for direct reimbursement by third-party payers "to advanced practice registered nurses who are practicing within their scope of practice under state law" (IOM, 2011, p. 10)

4. Modification of CMS hospital participation requirements for the Medicare program "to ensure that advanced practice registered nurses are eligible for clinical privileges, admitting privileges, and membership on medical staff" (IOM, 2011, p. 10)

5. Inclusion by the Office of Personnel Management for "coverage of those services of advanced practice registered nurses that are within their scope of practice under applicable state law" (IOM, 2011, p. 10)

6. Review of current and planned state regulations about APRNs by the Federal Trade Commission and the Antitrust Division of the Department of Justice "to identify those that have anticompetitive effects without contributing to the health and safety of the public" (IOM, 2011, p. 10)

The next section discusses progress in the first five years and the challenges affecting full practice, particularly for APRNs.

Build Common Ground around Scope of Practice and Other Issues in Policy & Practice (2015)

"Miss Nightingale was the founder of modern nursing because she made public opinion perceive, and act upon the perception, that nursing was an art, and must be raised to the status of a trained profession." —E. T. Cook (Cook, 1913a, p. 445)

"And I look upon it as a certainty that you will each be able, in one way or another to take a great part in reforming the Hospital and Workhouse Nursing systems of our country, perhaps of our colonies and dependencies, and perhaps of the world." —F. Nightingale (Nightingale, 2012, p. 47)

NIGHTINGALE'S VISION

Although "scope of practice" was not a term used in the Nightingale era, she realized that nursing practice must address policy issues to succeed. In 1866, Metropolitan workhouses (hospitals for the poor) were overcrowded and unsanitary. Pauper nurses were inadequate to deliver care to these patients. Nursing practice was to give medication to very ill patients three times a day and once daily to less ill patients. The nurse "poured out the medicine and judged according" (Cook, 1913b, p. 124). In 1867, the Metropolitan Poor Act was passed followed by a commission to improve medical relief in London workhouses. Florence Nightingale was the prime mover in this legislation. Her alliance with the Poor Law Inspector for the Metropolitan District pushed radical reform in workhouse nursing by recommending employment of competent nurses. Nightingale knew that the only way to workhouse reform was by reforming administration and finance. She also had to contend with a change in government administration from the Whig to the Tory party in 1866. Nightingale influenced public opinion, resulting in the Act of 1867, which was a foundation for improvements in medical relief and employment of trained nurses in these facilities. Her role was expressed by the Earl of Devon in the

House of Lords who stated, "It would be improper on such an occasion to omit reference to the improved feeling on the subject which had resulted from the admiration the country must feel for the exertions of that excellent and gifted woman, Miss Nightingale, whose name would always be received with that respect which was due to her Christian activity and self-devotion." (Cook, 1913b, p. 139).

Progress toward IOM's Vision

The Committee for Assessing Progress on Implementing the Recommendations of the Institute of Medicine report—*The Future of Nursing: Leading Change, Advancing Health*—was established in 2014 at the request of the Robert Wood Johnson Foundation (RWJF). In addition to assessing the progress of the 2010 IOM recommendations, this Study Committee's charge included identification of areas of focus for the next five years to meet these goals (National Academies of Sciences, Engineering, and Medicine, 2016).

Accomplishments

1. States in which APRNs can practice to the full extent of their education and license have increased since 2010. Per the recent Commission, eight additional states have granted full practice and prescriptive privileges to NPs, bringing the total of states with full practice authority to 21 (National Academies of Sciences, Engineering, and Medicine, 2016, p. 41). Other states have made legal improvements in their nurse practice acts with 17 states defined as reduced-practice and 12 as restricted-practice states (National Academies of Sciences, Engineering, and Medicine, 2016, p. 41). Note: The discrepancy can be explained by the use of different sources. Based on the figures of either document, progress has occurred in legislation granting full practice authority to APRNs.

2. Congress added a requirement by the ACA to the Public Health Service Act that prevents health insurers from denying covered services based on the provider's license (National Academies of Sciences, Engineering, and Medicine, 2016, p. 43).

3. A CMS final rule in 2012 allows hospitals to permit APRNs and other practitioners "to perform all functions within their scope of practice" (National Academies of Sciences, Engineering, and Medicine, 2016, p. 43).

4. A CMS final rule in 2014 "clarifies that outpatient services may be ordered by any practitioner, regardless of whether he or she is on a medical staff, if the practitioner is acting within his or her scope of practice under state law" (National Academies of Sciences, Engineering, and Medicine, 2016, p. 43).

5. The Federal Trade Commission (FTC) has actively pursued competition advocacy in many states to support APRNs' scope of practice and released a paper in 2014 expressing concern that physician supervision of nursing practice may limit patient access to APRNs (National Academies of Sciences, Engineering, and Medicine, 2016, p. 44).

6. The Veterans Health Administration (VHA) proposed independent practice for NPs employed by VHA in all states. A bill was introduced in 2015 in the U.S. Senate to grant full practice in VA facilities.
Note: In December 2016, the Department of Veterans Affairs granted full practice authority for APRNs within the scope of their employment except for Certified Registered Nurse Anesthetists (CRNAs) (38 CFR Part 17, Department of Veterans Affairs, 2016).

7. Both physicians and APRNs agree that additional nurse practitioners (NPs) would improve patient access to

care. There are also instances in which NPs' scope of practice is similar to physicians in some restricted-access states and supervision is not uniformly enforced. NPs and physicians are working collabora-tively on the grassroots level (National Academies of Sciences, Engineering, and Medicine, 2016).

Challenges

1. Despite the CMS rule of 2012, hospitals and state regulations continue to determine medical staff membership and hospital privileges (National Academies of Sciences, Engineering, and Medicine, 2016, p. 43).

2. Although the CMS rule of 2014 applies to all hospitals that participate in Medicare and Medicaid, individual hospitals have an option to restrict practice without penalty (National Academies of Sciences, Engineering, and Medicine, 2016, p. 43).

3. The American Medical Association (AMA), the American College of Physicians (ACA), and the Council of Medical Specialty Societies (CMSS) remain concerned about increasing the scope of practice for APRNs (National Academies of Sciences, Engineering, and Medicine, 2016, p. 46).

4. Shortages of primary care providers continue to exist in the United States (National Academies of Sciences, Engineering, and Medicine, 2016, p. 49).

Study Committee's Conclusion

"Continued work is needed to remove scope-of-practice barriers. The policy and practice context has shifted since *The Future of Nursing* was released. This shift has created an opportunity for nurses, physicians, and other providers to work together to find common ground in the new context of health care, and to devise solutions that work for all professions and patients" (National Academies of Sciences, Engineering, and Medicine, 2016, p. 51).

Study Committee's Recommendation

"The Future of Nursing: Campaign for Action (the Campaign) should broaden its coalition to include more diverse stakeholders. The Campaign should build on its successes and work with other health professions groups, policy makers, and the community to build common ground around removing scope-of-practice restrictions, increasing interprofessional collaboration, and addressing other issues to improve health care practice in the interest of patients (National Academies of Sciences, Engineering, and Medicine, 2016, pp. 51–52).

Nurses' Vision

What is your level of knowledge about the IOM (Institute of Medicine) recommendations for nursing?
This question established a baseline assessment for respondents. Responses included the following:

1. Know nothing about them = 36.21% (84 respondents)

2. Have skimmed the recommendations—minimal knowledge level = 39.22% (91 respondents)

3. Have read and understand the recommendations— competent knowledge level = 19.40% (45 respondents)

4. Involved in the implementation of the recommendations—expert knowledge level = 5.2% (12 respondents).

Are you able to practice to the limits of your license?
Yes = 88.26% (203 respondents)
No = 11.74% (27 respondents)

Comments

1. "The clinic I work in restricts scheduled drugs to the medical director. Given the circumstances of my clinic, I am OK with this policy, as it applies across the board to all providers (physicians, NPs, PAs, etc.)."

2. "Used nursing judgment necessary in last 18 years of practice. Less respect from physicians regarding nursing ability to assess, plan, and implement a plan independently from physician orders."

3. "My physical limitations prevent bedside care. The class you take in school falls on deaf ears because there is no context for practice. A class that educates a nurse about her license would have greater impact once the nurse has work experience and can apply their own experience/environment to standards."

4. "Cannot do ACLS at my facility."

5. "Unknown."

6. "Resources and processes limit the RN's ability to function at the top of their licensure. For example, nurses have to clean supplies and transport patients which takes time away from them coordinating the care plan or performing adequate patient education."

CHAPTER 3

Opportunities for Nurses to Lead and Diffuse Collaborative Improvement Efforts (2010)

"Miss Nightingale had for some time been in correspondence with Sir Henry Parkes, then Colonial Secretary in New South Wales, about the nursing in the Sydney Infirmary, and in December 1867, Miss Osburn sailed with five nurses to take up the position of Lady Superintendent . . . the diffusion of the Nightingale band did much to promote the extension of trained nursing in the Colony (Australia)."

—E. T. Cook
(Cook, 1913b, pp. 191–192)

"Valuable reports, replete with facts and suggestions drawn up by committees, inspectors, directors, and prefects, remain unknown to the public. Government ought to take care to make itself acquainted with, and promote the diffusion of all good methods, to watch all endeavours, to encourage every improvement. With our habits and institutions, there is but one instrument endowed with energy and power sufficient to secure this salutary influence—that instrument is the press."

—F. Nightingale (Cook, 1913a, p. 435)

NIGHTINGALE'S VISION

The Nightingale Training School evolved into a movement in which graduates became Lady Superintendents and Matrons in hospitals and other healthcare institutions throughout the world after recommendation by their Chief: Florence Nightingale. Hospitals in the United States were not immune from Nightingale's influence. Linda Richards who completed her postgraduate work at St. Thomas' Hospital, with Nightingale's encouragement returned to Boston and became the first Superintendent of Nurses at Massachusetts General Hospital (Cook, 1913a, p. 465; Judd, Sitzman, & Davis, 2010, p. 41). Miss Alice Fisher who revitalized Blockley Hospital in Philadelphia, was another graduate of the Nightingale School (Cook, 1913a, p. 465). Matrons and Superintendents improved care delivery, and some founded training schools for nurses in their new communities. The placement and advancement to pivotal leadership positions did not occur by accident. Nightingale maintained close contact with these nurse leaders, providing timely advice and communication regardless of their location. She realized that collaboration with organization leaders (committees) was essential for success of superintendents and matrons.

For example, when a Matron had a disagreement with her committee and considered resigning her position, Nightingale advised her, "Is not the thing of first importance to lay a statement of the whole case before your President? Nay, would it not be breaking faith with him if it were not done? This *is* now being done. Is not the next thing for you to take no step till you know the results of this letter to him—the next action he will take? You will remember that I stated to him at your friend's suggestion and at yours, that you wished for, that you *invited, a full investigation to be made by him and that you wished to abide by his decision.* I thought this so important, in order that I might not appear to be asking for any personal favour but only for justice, that I underlined it. Will it not seem as if you were afraid to await his full understanding of the case (how far from the truth!) if you precipitately resigned before he had had time even to consider the statement? The Matron must show no fear, else it would indeed be sacrificing the fruit of eight years' most excellent work. Surely she should wait quietly— that is the true dignity—with her friends around her till the President's answer is given. The 'persecuted for righteousness sake' never run away" (Cook, 1913b, pp. 261–262).

Nightingale set an example for her nurses in leading and diffusing collaborative efforts. She maintained a wide circle of advisors and professional colleagues who collaborated with her to achieve lofty goals to improve health. For example, she began corresponding with a Liverpool philanthropist in 1861 about beginning a system of district nursing there to provide better care to the poor. Because there were no trained nurses in Liverpool, Nightingale suggested starting a training school in the Royal Infirmary there. The school started in 1862 with guidance from Nightingale and became a success. The philanthropist and Nightingale then collaborated to improve the Workhouse Infirmary in Liverpool. She arranged for 12 Nightingale nurses to be employed there and selected a Lady Superintendent. That choice was critical for the project's success. Miss Agnes Jones, an outstanding St. Thomas' graduate, accepted the position after interviewing with Nightingale. It was a formidable undertaking. There were 1,200 patients living in filthy conditions being cared for by untrained and pauper nurses. Agnes Jones and the 12 Nightingale nurses faced a daunting task. She terminated 35 nurses in the first few months for drunkenness. The philanthropist and Miss Jones didn't always agree, and disputes were negotiated with Nightingale playing a significant role in resolution. Miss Jones found a better approach to getting things done when dealing with the officials of the organization. She suggested changes that weren't accepted by the officials. She allowed a decent interval to elapse and planted the seed so that the officials made the same suggestion. Then, she stated that those suggestions were excellent and changes evolved. It was a slower, but highly effective process. The success of the Liverpool experiment encouraged Nightingale to pursue a similar approach in London. She began by collecting data about all London infirmaries. Then, she worked with representatives of both political parties to achieve legislation to improve London workhouses. It was a good beginning, but she knew that the struggle would go on, and her writings and collaboration with political leaders were augmented by her letter to the *Times* that made the Metropolitan Nursing Association well known to the public. One of Nightingale's best pupils, Miss Florence Lees, was appointed as Lady Superintendent on her recommendation to successfully organize district nursing in London. According to Nightingale, this system in London was "twenty years ago a paradox, but twenty years hence will be a commonplace" (Cook, 1913b, p. 253). Her words were prophetic.

IOM'S VISION

"Private and public funders, health care organizations, nursing education programs, and nursing associations should expand opportunities for nurses to lead and manage collaborative efforts with physicians and other members of the health care team to conduct research and to redesign and improve practice environments and health systems. These entities should also provide opportunities for nurses to diffuse successful practices" (IOM, 2011, p. 11).

The changing health care environment requires nurses, physicians, and other health professionals to collaborate as an interprofessional team to achieve quality and safe patient care. The Committee realized that nurses were frequently seen as followers rather than leaders in decision making. Nurses, particularly staff nurses, had crucial knowledge about patient and community needs based on their skills, education, and experience. However, they were often reluctant to express their ideas and concerns and relied on direction from physicians and others.

Leadership competencies for nurses must include initial skills (e.g., knowledge of care delivery system, teamwork, collaboration, ethics, advocacy, quality, and safety, etc.) and advanced skills (e.g., full partnership in an interprofessional team, holding self and others accountable, knowledge of payment systems, regulatory issues, impact of economic forces on health care, etc.) (IOM, 2011, pp. 223–224).

Nurses at all levels must be leaders who know when to collaborate, intercede, advocate, defer to other leaders, or step up to lead the team. The ACA offered opportunities for nurses at all levels—students, staff nurses, community health nurses, chief nursing officers, members of nursing organizations, and researchers—to attain leadership competencies and serve as leaders in interprofessional collaboration with other health team members (IOM, 2011, p. 251).

Nurses' leadership development takes many forms. The most common approach is formal leadership training programs. Many of these programs are geared toward nurses in leadership and executive positions. Mentorship by other nurses, other health professionals, and business leaders provides guidance and opportunities for professional growth by sharing expertise and support. Involvement in political action and policy development is an opportunity for nurses to lead in improving quality and patient access to care (IOM, 2011, pp. 241–245).

IOM's supporting recommendations included the following:

1. Support by the Center for Medicare and Medicaid Innovation (CMMI) for models of care delivery and reimbursement that employ nurses as leaders to reduce costs and improve outcomes. Nurses' contributions to best practices should be reflected in performance measures (IOM, 2011, p. 11).

2. Funding for research by private and public payers about care models and innovations that empower

nurses to impact health care improvements (IOM, 2011, p. 11).

3. Support by health care organizations for nurses to lead in creating and implementing patient-focused, innovative care models (IOM, 2011, p. 11).

4. Support by health care organizations for involvement of nurses and other staff members to collaborate "with developers and manufacturers in the design, development, purchase, implementation, and evaluation of medical and health devices and health information technology products" (IOM, 2011, p. 11).

5. Provision of professional development programs by nursing associations and education programs to foster nurse-led "programs and businesses that will contribute to improved health and health care" (IOM, 2011, p. 11).

The next section describes progress toward nurse leadership in interprofessional collaboration to advance patient-focused care in the five years after the IOM Report and future implications.

Expand Efforts and Opportunities for Interprofessional Collaboration and Leadership for Nurses (2015)

"There is no magic in the word 'Association,' but there is a secret, a mighty call in it, *if* we will but listen to the 'still small voice' in it, calling upon each of us to do our best. We might never forget that the 'Individual' makes the

Association. What the Association *is* depends upon each of its members. A Nurses' Association can never be a substitute for the individual Nurse. It is she who must, each in her measure, give life to the Association, while the Association helps *her*." —F. Nightingale (Nightingale, 2012, p. 140)

NIGHTINGALE'S VISION

Nightingale expanded efforts and opportunities for interprofessional collaboration and leadership throughout her life. In 1888, County Councils were created by law in England. In 1889, these councils could collect taxes and spend money on technical education. The Local Taxation Act of 1890 provided significant funding from the "Whiskey Money" (Cook, 1913b, p. 383). Funds were available and the definition of technical education was broad. Nightingale collaborated with Frederick Verney, the chairman of the North Bucks' Technical Education Committee to develop women health missioners for that district to provide education information to people in their own homes. It was a novel idea and they collaborated with the District Health Officer to conduct the training of these women. That physician used lectures and classes as well as practical experiences in district villages to share health information with his students. They were required to pass an examination and complete a probationary period in the role before being certified as Health Missioners. After certification, some were employed by the North Bucks' Technical Education Committee to present health education in the villages. Nightingale's leadership role included recruiting applicants, collecting best practice information about sanitary education, and evaluating examination content and syllabi. Her extensive research on the subject included correspondence with other technical education committees, resulting in her paper on rural hygiene presented at the Women Workers' Conference at Leeds in November 1893. The pilot project spread through other technical education committees. Nightingale's leadership and interprofessional collaboration with the District Health Officer was successful in providing health education and sanitary instruction by qualified, trained health missioners in rural England (Cook, 1913b, p. 384).

Progress toward IOM's Vision

The Study Committee reviewed progress toward the goal for nurses to lead and disseminate collaborative improvement activities five years after publication of the IOM Report.

Accomplishments

1. Interprofessional collaboration is part of the curriculum for accredited baccalaureate, master's, and doctoral nursing education (National Academies of Sciences, Engineering, and Medicine, 2016, p. 138).

2. The Commission on Collegiate Nursing Education (CCNE) has allied with five health professions' accrediting bodies—medicine, pharmacy, dentistry, osteopathy, and public health—to partner and develop competencies and curricula for interprofessional education (National Academies of Sciences, Engineering, and Medicine, 2016, p. 139).

3. The Interprofessional Education Collaboration (IPEC) developed core competencies for interprofessional collaborative practice in 2011 (National Academies of Sciences, Engineering, and Medicine, 2016, p. 140).

4. CMMI created the Health Care Innovation Awards that financially reward organizations whose projects reduce costs and improve health. Nurses are leaders or interprofessional team members for several of these projects (National Academies of Sciences, Engineering, and Medicine, 2016, p. 140).

5. The Health Resources and Services Administration (HRSA) provided more than $67 million from 2012 to 2014 for interprofessional collaborative practice (National Academies of Sciences, Engineering, and Medicine, 2016, pp. 140–141).

6. Many organizations are acting to increase interprofessional practice (National Academies of Sciences, Engineering, and Medicine, 2016, p. 141).

7. Twenty-five State Action Coalitions are focusing on models for interprofessional practice or education (National Academies of Sciences, Engineering, and Medicine, 2016, pp. 141–142).

8. Interprofessional education continues to expand at nursing schools (National Academies of Sciences, Engineering, and Medicine, 2016, p. 142).

Challenges

1. Interprofessional education must expand beyond simulation and conferences in acute care settings to encompass community sites (National Academies of Sciences, Engineering, and Medicine, 2016, p. 139).

2. Support for interprofessional education will require a cultural change for acceptance by older physicians (National Academies of Sciences, Engineering, and Medicine, 2016, p. 139).

3. The Campaign's only metric for interprofessional education focuses on required courses/activities at the top 10 nursing schools with "both registered nurse (RN) students and other graduate health professional students" (National Academies of Sciences, Engineering, and Medicine, 2016, p. 142).

4. New models of care must employ registered nurses as team leaders or facilitators with all interprofessional team members unified to benefit the patient (National Academies of Sciences, Engineering, and Medicine, 2016, p. 144).

5. Leadership development is essential for all members of Interprofessional teams (National Academies of Sciences, Engineering, and Medicine, 2016, p. 155).

6. The State Action Coalitions need to include more stakeholders to continue progress on nurses' participation and leadership in interprofessional collaboration (National Academies of Sciences, Engineering, and Medicine, 2016, p. 145).

Progress has been made on interprofessional education and collaboration in the past five years. More work must occur to achieve nursing leadership within teams that are based on mutual respect and are united in providing patient-focused care in today's health care environment (National Academies of Sciences, Engineering, and Medicine, 2016).

Study Committee's Conclusion

"True interprofessional collaboration can be accomplished only in concert with other health professionals, not within the nursing profession alone. State Action Coalitions need assistance in reaching out to non-nursing stakeholders. In the new context of health care, the Campaign itself needs to be a broader coalition of stakeholders from all health care professions if it is to make progress" (National Academies of Sciences, Engineering, and Medicine, 2016, p. 145).

Study Committee's Recommendation

"As the Campaign broadens its coalition, it should expand its focus on supporting and promoting (1) interprofessional collaboration and opportunities for nurses to design, implement, and diffuse collaborative programs in care and delivery; and (2) interdisciplinary development programs that focus on leadership. Health care professionals from all disciplines should work together in the planning and implementation of strategies for improving health care, particularly in an interprofessional and collaborative environment" (National Academies of Sciences, Engineering, and Medicine, 2016, p. 155).

Nurses' Vision

Do you lead interprofessional (involving other professions and nursing) collaborative improvement projects?

1. Yes = 32.47% (75 respondents)

2. No = 67.53% (156 respondents)

Comments

1. "I work casual in a nursing home."

2. "Participated in some committees."

3. "I do participate and actively seek to participate."

4. "Only when I was a BSN student. I precepted with the Trauma Department and created their Fall Prevention Program that they used for their ACS (American College of Surgeons) trauma survey that involved other professions and the community."

5. "Nurse residents and family practice/internal medicine medical residents complete SIM (simulation) cases together to practice communication skills."

6. "Leadership needs to make this more of a priority and identify 'champions' that can work together to advance competence related to the core competencies for interprofessional collaborative practice."

7. "I worked with the director of lab to help change practice in the ED regarding the use of rainbow tubes of blood being drawn. She led the team and was instrumental in saving $62,000.00 a year."

8. "No, we had committees at one point. I was on a patient education committee. But being part of a corporation, we work to the points sent down from corporate. Which leaves little time for additional education interventions—including important things like medication information when sending patients home. Also night shift is excluded from meetings held at 9 or 10 am. Scheduling them later in the day and keeping up the patient information folders would make discharge process smoother, and everyone would be better informed as to what they need to do. So simple, but so hard to accomplish!"

9. "All nurses have skills that they are an expert at and others that they are proficient. I have been working with ortho/neuro/trauma staff to have those that have an identified weakness get to be content experts and coach others on the unit. The bedside nurses are helping me instruct on the unit level. It empowers and teaches leadership skills."

CHAPTER 4

Implement Nurse Residency Programs (2010)

"Training 'consists in teaching people to bear responsibilities, and laying the responsibilities on them as they are able to bear them,' as Bishop Patteson said of Education."

—F. Nightingale
(Nightingale, 2012, p. 106)

Florence Nightingale knew that graduates of the Nightingale School would be employed in many different nursing positions and that they must be oriented to their responsibilities. Although nurse residency programs did not exist at that time, she served as a mentor and preceptor for her nurses through regular written communication and their periodic visits to her home. Her volume of correspondence increased over the years and her advice, support, and encouragement enabled the nurses to accept and meet challenges. According to her biographer, "I have counted as many as a hundred letters received in a year from a single Superintendent. There were several years in which the total of Miss Nightingale's nursing correspondence has to be counted in thousands" (Cook, 1913b, p. 262). Her wisdom and common sense was reflected in these letters to inform and advance her protégées as shown in her advice to a candidate for a nursing position to avoid beginning employment by seeking "to reform the whole system" (Cook, 1913b, p. 259). Nightingale's approach to postgraduate development and integration in their care delivery settings was successful when there were no formal residency programs.

IOM'S VISION

"State boards of nursing, accrediting bodies, the federal government, and health care organizations should take actions to support nurses' completion of a transition-to-practice program (nurse residency) after they have completed a prelicensure or advanced practice degree program or when they are transitioning into new clinical practice areas" (IOM, 2011, p. 11).

As early as 2002, The Joint Commission (TJC) recommended nurse residency programs for graduates to "acquire the knowledge and skills to deliver safe, quality care that meets defined (organization or society) standards of practice" (IOM, 2011, pp. 120–121). The Committee explored high turnover rates in nurse graduates related to inadequate transition to practice. A troubling issue was nurses who left the profession after quitting their first position (IOM, 2011).

The Committee examined data on the cost and effectiveness of nurse residency programs, including reduction of first-year turnover. These residency programs—Versant, the University HealthSystem Consortium (UHC), and the American Association of Colleges of Nursing (AACN)— have been primarily employed in acute care health care facilities. The ACA demonstrated the need for skilled nurses in community settings outside acute care. The Committee investigated nurse residencies in nonacute care settings.

Such programs are called mentoring programs, internships, or orientation programs. Their purpose is to provide structured opportunities to gain a deeper understanding of population health through experiences in community and home settings. Participants attain competencies through mentoring and hands-on activities over a three- to six-month orientation. Such programs focus on recruiting and retaining nurses (IOM, 2011, p. 122). The Committee determined that such non-acute care residencies are not universal and must increase to meet the needs of new nurses and the goals of these agencies.

Most evidence about successful nurse residency programs has come from programs' self-evaluations. Such evaluations described significant turnover savings, increased retention rates, more stable staffing levels, improved skills and satisfaction of first-year nurses, and return on investment for the organization. The Committee concentrated on new nurse residencies because of available data, but recognized the need for residencies for experienced nurses transitioning to new areas in acute or community care. They believed that APRNs could benefit from a residency after completing their graduate education. The Committee also recommended that nurses be paid during residency programs in either acute or community care but did not take a position on whether salary should be full or reduced. They stated that educational debt and loans should not be repaid during the residency programs (IOM, 2011, pp. 123–124).

Specific recommendations included the following:

1. Accrediting bodies and state boards of nursing should collaborate to support nurse residency completion after completion of an undergraduate or advanced practice nursing program as well as during transition to new clinical areas (IOM, 2011, p. 12).

2. The Secretary of Health and Human Services (HHS) should reassign "all graduate medical education

funding from diploma nursing programs to support the implementation of nurse residency programs in rural or critical access areas" (IOM, 2011, p. 12).

3. HRSA, CMS, health care organizations, and philanthropic organizations should finance "the development and implementation of nurse residency programs across all practice settings" (IOM, 2011, p. 12).

4. Nurse residency programs should be evaluated for effectiveness in improving nurses' retention, increasing competencies, and improvement of patient outcomes by their health care organizations and foundations (IOM, 2011, p. 12).

What is the status of nurse residency programs for new RN graduates, experienced nurses transitioning to new clinical settings, and APRNs five years after the IOM recommendations? That is examined in the next section.

Create and Fund Transition-to-Practice Programs (2015)

"Miss Nightingale formulated a scheme. The Committee of her Council met the Governors of the Hospital, and an agreement was arrived at for the foundation of the Nightingale School. The basis of the agreement was that the Hospital was to provide facilities for the training, and the Nightingale Fund to pay the cost, including the payment of the nurses themselves. Thus on a modest scale, but with a vast amount of forethought, was launched the scheme which was destined to found the modern art and practice of nursing." —E. T. Cook (Cook, 1913a, p. 459)

Transition-to-practice programs were not available in the Nightingale era. Funding the first nurse training school in England was an opportunity that enabled Florence Nightingale to change nursing from a haven for drunks and prostitutes to a profession of educated women of high ideals. This opportunity only transpired due to her service in the Crimea. Her achievements were published in the *Times*, and the people of England—royals and commoners alike—were captivated by this gentlewoman's exploits. As her legend grew, Nightingale became ill from nursing patients with Crimean fever. As she recovered, she refused to return home and the British people wanted to honor her heroism and recognize her service. The resulting Nightingale Fund enabled her to design, establish, and direct a school to train nurses. Although championed by many, the Fund was not universally supported. Lord Granville wrote "Lady Pam thinks the Nightingale Fund great humbug. 'The nurses are very good now; perhaps they do drink a little, but so do the ladies' monthly nurses, and nothing can be better than them; poor people, it must be so tiresome sitting up all night.'" (Cook, 1913a, pp. 272–273). Luckily for Nightingale and the future of nursing, her sentiments did not prevail. The Fund grew with contributions by soldiers as well as people from all walks of life. On June 24, 1860, the Nightingale Training School for Nurses finally opened at St. Thomas' Hospital in London. She established a Council of distinguished Englishmen to manage the trusts created for the Nightingale Fund, which had grown to £44,000. After reviewing numerous hospitals and charities, she chose St. Thomas' Hospital because it was well-managed and had a Matron of remarkable administrative and nursing ability. The agreement provided facilities for training nurses, and the Fund paid the cost, including a stipend for the nurse probationers. The initial class had 15 probationers in the one-year training program. It was a modest start, but Nightingale had planned well for this transition to modern nursing. She realized that her training school would be a template for others and the Fund enabled her to prepare and position her graduates to advance nursing and healthcare in multiple settings and countries (Cook, 1913a).

Progress toward IOM's Vision

The Study Committee agreed with the IOM findings that residencies are beneficial for both new nursing graduates and APRNs on completion of their graduate education. They also concluded that residency programs in community and outpatient settings have not received enough attention.

Accomplishments

1. The National Council of State Boards of Nursing began studying models for transition to practice by nurse graduates in multiple settings—hospitals, home care, long-term care, etc.—in 2011 (National Academies of Sciences, Engineering, and Medicine, 2016, p. 6).

2. Transition-to-practice nurse residencies have had positive outcomes: better organizational, time management, and communication skills by participants and improved retention (National Academies of Sciences, Engineering, and Medicine, 2016, pp. 6–7).

Challenges

1. Data is inadequate to evaluate the success of nurse residency programs (National Academies of Sciences, Engineering, and Medicine, 2016, p. 7).

2. Nurse residency programs are variable (National Academies of Sciences, Engineering, and Medicine, 2016, p. 7).

3. It is difficult to determine growth of overall programs in diverse health care settings, and for nurses with different educational levels (National Academies of Sciences, Engineering, and Medicine, 2016, p. 7).

4. The cost of nurse residency programs is a barrier to wider implementation (National Academies of Sciences, Engineering, and Medicine, 2016, p. 7).

Study Committee's Conclusion

"This committee believes that residencies for both RNs and APRNs are beneficial and need to be encouraged and that attention to residency programs for outpatient care is insufficient" (National Academies of Sciences, Engineering, and Medicine, 2016, p. 7).

Study Committee's Recommendation

"The Campaign, in coordination with health care providers, health care delivery organizations, and payers, should lead efforts to explore ways of creating and funding transition-to-practice residency programs at both the registered nurse and advanced practice registered nurse levels. Such programs are needed in all practice settings, including community-based practices and long-term care. These efforts should include determining the most appropriate program models; setting standards for programs; exploring funding and business case models; and creating an overarching structure with which to track and evaluate the quality, effectiveness, and impact of transition-to-practice programs" (National Academies of Sciences, Engineering, and Medicine, 2016, p. 8).

Nurses' Vision

Does your healthcare setting have a transition-to-practice residency for new RNs?

1. Yes = 63.56% (145 respondents)

2. No = 36.44% (82 respondents)

Comments

1. "Unfortunately, our residency is a theory-based initiative. It is not certified and because it is currently a research project, changes are not made based on new graduate feedback. Funding is out of individual nursing unit budgets. It is a step in the right direction, but we have a LONG way to go!"

2. "Yes—the Versant program, about 18 weeks for new graduates. I went through this two years ago and all from my cohort are still employed at the hospital, but several of us changed units of care. We do follow-up 'metrics' yearly. The overall feeling from traditionally-trained nurses seems to be that a residency is just 'hand-holding' and that 'sink or swim' is the way to go. They voice that the resident nurses are no more capable than a nonresident nurse, but as all new grads are coming on board through the Versant program, there are less complaints."

3. "Yes for RNs → months. We are still collecting data. It is a 'home-grown' program utilizing volunteers or free resources. We utilize BKAT and Casey-Fink assessments for evaluation. It is not certified."

4. "Not sure."

5. "Don't know." (×2)

6. "Critical care units do."

7. "Occasionally. I was a part of the FIRST new grad ICU residency at my hospital. It was a one-time occurrence for ICU, and they did a one-time program for the ED."

8. "I work in pharma."

9. "I work in an office where RN experience is a prerequisite."

10. "Yes, but it is an awful waste of time. I was miserable every minute."

11. "Work in home hospice—new RNs not hired, experience required."

12. "We used to—recently eliminated the program :((sad face.)"

13. "No. They (residents) need to be helped in the project that they complete so that it involves EBP or research. Everyone knows how to do QI. No one wants to take the time to do an EBP or research project."

Does your healthcare setting have a fellowship program for advanced practice nurses?

1. Yes = 16.67% (35 respondents)

2. No = 83.33% (175 respondents)

Comments

1. "Unsure." (×10)

2. "Will be implementing a succession planning fellowship for nurse leaders in 2017."

3. "Just beginning."

4. "I don't know." (×4)

5. "I work in pharma."

6. "NA."

7. "No program for ARNPs."

CHAPTER 5

Increase Proportion of Nurses with a Baccalaureate Degree to 80% by 2020 (2010)

"For us who Nurse, our Nursing is a thing, which, unless in it we are making progress every year, every month, every week, take my word for it we are going back. A woman who thinks in herself: 'Now, I am a "full" Nurse, a "skilled" Nurse, I have learnt all that there is to be learnt': take my word for it, she does not know *what a Nurse is*, and she never *will* know; she is *gone* back already."

—F. Nightingale
(Nightingale, 2012, p. 1)

NIGHTINGALE'S VISION

Florence Nightingale's own formal nursing education was limited to three months residence in 1851 at the Institution for Deaconesses in Kaiserwerth, Germany. Kaiserwerth was founded by Pastor Theodor Fliedner and contained a 100-bed hospital, an infant school, a penitentiary, and a normal school. Of the 116 deaconesses, 94 were consecrated by receiving a blessing in church. The others were probationers. The training for nurses was meager, but patients were not neglected. Food was inferior, but the environment was clean, and the staff was devoted to their charges. She spent two weeks there a year earlier and, in 1853, went to Paris to study with the Sisters of Charity and learn in their hospitals. She inspected other hospitals and infirmaries and analyzed their statistics about hospital and nursing care. Unfortunately, her grandmother became terminally ill, and she had to return home before starting her apprenticeship in Paris. The limits of her formal nursing education inspired Nightingale to provide high-quality training for nurses at the Nightingale School years later (Cook, 1913a).

Although degrees were not awarded, her vision created the modern profession of nursing. That was a singular achievement that positively impacts our practice today.

IOM'S VISION

"Nurses should achieve higher levels of education and training through an improved education system that promotes seamless academic progression" (IOM, 2011, p. 163).

Several different pathways exist to become a nurse. Licensed practical nurses (LVNs/LPNs) are prepared in vocational programs to provide essential patient care in long-term care settings. Their education program encompasses both technical and nursing skills. Education options preparing registered nurses include diploma schools, associate degree

(AD) programs, and bachelor of science in nursing (BSN) programs (IOM, 2011, pp. 165–166).

Because few diploma programs still exist, many students obtain an Associate Degree in Nursing through two years of study (if the student can obtain all required courses in that length of time) in a community college. A Bachelor of Science in Nursing degree is a four-year degree that includes liberal arts, advanced sciences, leadership development, and public health clinical experience along with nursing courses and hospital experiences (IOM, 2011, p. 166).

Graduates of these three education programs are eligible to take the same licensing exam (NCLEX-RN) to validate their "minimum competency required to practice nursing safely" (IOM, 2011, p. 167). The exam is geared toward acute care settings because that is where most new graduates have worked in the past. The Committee realized that, as health care moves into community settings, NCLEX content must change to reflect applicable competencies for competent practice beyond acute care (IOM, 2011, pp. 167–168).

The Committee determined that the BSN degree should become the entry level-degree for registered nurses because it provides a wider variety of competencies that nurses will need as they lead care coordination activities. Health care is complex universally and nurses with additional education will be better equipped to handle these challenges. Shortages of BSN-prepared registered nurses presented an obstacle to nursing care coordination (IOM, 2011, p. 170).

However, they also realized that nursing education is costly and that many students lack financial resources to obtain BSN degrees, starting with ADNs first and progressing to BSNs when they can afford the costs. Different pathways are available for nurses to achieve the BSN including traditional RN-to-BSN programs, employee tuition assistance programs, collaboration between hospitals and local colleges, collaboration between community colleges and universities, online courses, and new curriculum models (IOM, 2011, pp. 173–174).

The Committee advocated phasing out diploma schools within 10 years by consolidating their courses with community colleges or university programs and using their federal funding support to grow baccalaureate nursing programs and higher nursing education programs. Because BSN-prepared registered nurses will not reach 100% in a short time, the Committee set a goal of 80% by 2020 (IOM, 2011, pp. 173–174). They understood that four barriers must be addressed for nursing education to have capacity that meets the educational needs of undergraduate students. These barriers are the following:

1. There is a shortage of qualified nursing faculty, and many of these are older (IOM, 2011, p. 179).

2. There are insufficient clinical placement opportunities to ensure that students attain competencies to function effectively postgraduation (IOM, 2011, p. 189).

3. There is a need for curriculum changes that include competencies to meet the need of future patients in all settings and prepare nurses for higher degrees (IOM, 2011, pp. 190–191).

4. Inadequate workforce planning doesn't align market demands with educational capacity and affects each level of nursing education (IOM, 2011, p. 179).

Supporting recommendations included the following:

1. All nursing schools should be required "to offer defined academic pathways, beyond articulation

agreements, that promote seamless access for nurses to higher levels of education" (IOM, 2011, p. 12).

2. Health care organizations should support nurses in entering BSN programs within five years' post-graduation "by offering tuition reimbursement, creating a culture that fosters continuing education, and providing a salary differential and promotion" (IOM, 2011, p. 12).

3. Funders, both public and private, should work together to ensure the growth of students in BSN programs "by offering scholarships and loan forgiveness, hiring more faculty, expanding clinical instruction through new clinical partnerships, and using technology to augment instruction" (IOM, 2011, p. 12).

4. Federal and state agencies and private funders should "expand loans and grants for second-degree nursing students" (IOM, 2011, p. 13).

5. Nursing and other health professional schools "should design and implement early and continuous interprofessional collaboration through joint classroom and clinical training opportunities" (IOM, 2011, p. 13).

6. "Academic nurse leaders should partner with health care organizations, leaders from primary and secondary school systems, and other community organizations to recruit and advance diverse nursing students" (IOM, 2011, p. 13).

How successful have these initiatives been in the past five years to move the percentage of BSN-prepared registered nurses to 80% by 2020? That is addressed in the next section.

Continue Pathways toward Increasing the Percentage of Nurses with a Baccalaureate Degree (2015)

"The more experience we gain, the more progress we can make. The progress you make in your year's training with us is as nothing to what you must make every year *after* your year's training is over." —F. Nightingale (Nightingale, 2012, p. 1)

Many founders would have resented the inception of other nurse training schools, but Florence Nightingale welcomed them. She considered them alternate pathways to increase the number and proficiency of trained nurses. Several of these schools were developed and led by Nightingale nurses. Examples included training schools at Edinburgh Hospital, the Marylebone Infirmary, St. Mary's Hospital, and Westminster Hospital (Cook, 1913b, p. 256). Their graduates amplified the scope of Nightingale's vision of nursing education in sites nationally and internationally. When her probationers at the Nightingale School expressed concern about the development of additional training schools, she succinctly expressed her feelings by saying, "Let us hail the successes of other Training Schools, sprung up, thank God, so fast and well in latter years. But the best way we can hail them is not to be left behind ourselves. Let us, in the spirit of friendly rivalry, rejoice in their progress, as they do, I am sure, in ours. *All* can win the prize. One training school is not lowered because others win. On the contrary, all are lowered if others fail" (Cook, 1913b, p. 257). Nightingale's behavior demonstrated the truth of her words. She was helpful and supportive of these pathways to move nursing forward as a profession.

Progress toward IOM's Vision

Per the Study Committee, it will be problematic to achieve the IOM goal of 80% baccalaureate-prepared registered nurses by 2020. However, progress has occurred in the number of undergraduate entry-level and fast-track baccalaureate programs as well as completion programs for licensed registered nurses (National Academies of Sciences, Engineering, and Medicine, 2016).

Accomplishments

1. The Robert Wood Johnson Foundation has funded the Academic Progression in Nursing program managed by the Tri-Council for Nursing to help states and localities develop plans for "academic progression and baccalaureate-prepared nurse employment" (National Academies of Sciences, Engineering, and Medicine, 2016, pp. 59–60).

2. The New Mexico Education Consortium (NMNEC) has developed a common curriculum to provide a seamless transfer between community colleges and universities. State funded schools offering ADNs and BSNs adopted this model in 2012. Students can remain in their communities and finish their baccalaureate program online or in clinical experiences (National Academies of Sciences, Engineering, and Medicine, 2016, pp. 60–61).

3. Pre- and postlicensure baccalaureate degree programs have increased in the five years after the IOM report was published (National Academies of Sciences, Engineering, and Medicine, 2016, pp. 63–65).

4. Employers and market forces indicate a preference for BSN-prepared registered nurses (National Academies of Sciences, Engineering, and Medicine, 2016, p. 68).

5. Research evidence shows that hospitals with a higher percentage of BSNs have better patient outcomes resulting in cost savings (National Academies of Sciences, Engineering, and Medicine, 2016, p. 71).

6. Since 2012, the number of baccalaureate-prepared registered nurses has continued to exceed the number of associate degree registered nurses (National Academies of Sciences, Engineering, and Medicine, 2016, p. 66).

Challenges

1. HRSA funding for loans and grants for nursing education programs has not increased (National Academies of Sciences, Engineering, and Medicine, 2016, p. 66).

2. Full data about loan funding by states and private funders for nursing education programs is not readily available (National Academies of Sciences, Engineering, and Medicine, 2016, p. 67).

3. Most employers do not require a BSN for employment (National Academies of Sciences, Engineering, and Medicine, 2016, p. 68).

4. Nursing schools reject qualified applicants for BSN programs due to "faculty shortages, a lack of clinical sites or classroom space, and budget constraints" (National Academies of Sciences, Engineering, and Medicine, 2016, p. 71).

5. Barriers identified by nurses "include financial concerns; a lack of time and competing priorities; logistical concerns; a lack of academic support; and a perceived lack of clinical, professional, or economic value in a higher degree" (National Academies of Sciences, Engineering, and Medicine, 2016, p. 71).

6. Hospital incentives for baccalaureate nursing education are not universal or available in nonacute care settings (National Academies of Sciences, Engineering, and Medicine, 2016, p. 71).

7. The quality of new BSN-completion programs must be validated (National Academies of Sciences, Engineering, and Medicine, 2016, p. 72).

Study Committee's Conclusion

"Between 2010 and 2014, the proportion of employed nurses with a baccalaureate degree or higher in nursing increased from 49 percent to 51 percent" (National Academies of Sciences, Engineering, and Medicine, 2016, p. 73).

Study Committee's Recommendation

Market forces are increasingly favoring baccalaureate-prepared nurses, particularly in hospital settings. As the RN population shifts to becoming increasingly baccalaureate-prepared, unintended consequences with respect to the employment, earning power, skills, and roles and responsibilities of those nurses who do not achieve higher education may occur" (National Academies of Sciences, Engineering, and Medicine, 2016, p. 74).

Make Diversity in the Workforce a Priority (2015)

"I do not feel though Pagan in the morning, Jew in the afternoon, and Christian in the evening, anything but a unity of interest in all these representations. To know God we must study Him as much in the Pagan and Jewish dispensations as in the Christian . . . and this gives unity to the whole—one continuous thread of interest to all these pearls." —F. Nightingale (Cook, 1913a, p. 74)

"My Committee (in her first position at Harley Street) refused me to take in *Catholic* patients—whereupon I wished them good morning, unless I might take in Jews and their Rabbis. So now it is settled . . . that we are to take in all denominations whatever, and allow them to be visited by their respective priests and Muftis . . ."
—F. Nightingale (Cook, 1913a, p. 134)

NIGHTINGALE'S VISION

Florence Nightingale's vision related to diversity focused on the inclusion of women nurses in military hospitals. Sisters of nursing orders in other countries fulfilled this role, but England had not authorized this approach when the Crimean War began in 1854. There was a stark contrast between care that French soldiers in the Crimea received from the Sisters of Charity and Sisters of Mercy and the lack of attention to the needs of injured English soldiers. The *Times* correspondent in Constantinople alerted the public to these deficiencies through a series of published letters. A letter published on October 14 would have profound effects on the role of women as nurses in military hospitals and on Nightingale's role in making this workforce diversity a priority. The letter stated, "Why have we no Sisters of Charity? There are numbers of able-bodied and tender-hearted English women who would joyfully and with alacrity go out to devote themselves to nursing the sick and wounded, if they could be associated for that purpose, and placed under proper protection" (Cook, 1918a, p. 148). Sidney Herbert, Secretary at War, served as representative for the Secretary of State about these hospitals and knew that good intentions were not enough to introduce women as nurses in military hospitals in the war zone. He realized that only one English nurse was capable of succeeding in the role of Superintendent of female nurses in the Crimea: Florence Nightingale. After she accepted the position, Nightingale began to vet candidates for this mission. That was an arduous task because few trained nurses were available outside the religious sisterhoods.

Nightingale was aware of the delicacy of her position. Gender diversity presented numerous difficulties, and her approach was carefully planned. She aligned herself with the Commander, Lord Raglan, who provided essential support for her task. Outwardly, military officers were polite, but some tried to undermine her activities. Nightingale remained calm under tremendous pressure and gained support from most physicians by her efficiency and effectiveness. She diplomatically introduced her nurses into this complex environment while maintaining discipline among them. As one nurse stated, "Miss Nightingale told us only to attend to patients in the wards of those surgeons who wished for our services, and she charged us never to do anything for the patients without the leave of the doctors (Cook, 1913a, p. 182). She

gained support from medical leaders and the Senior Chaplain. Most of all, she was loved by the soldiers (Cook, 1913a).

Nightingale's success in the Crimea opened the door to women nurses in military hospitals. She always supported their presence and encouraged their success. In 1882, 24 women nurses, including several graduates of the Nightingale School, served in the Egyptian Campaign. They communicated regularly with Nightingale, who encouraged them and cheered their accomplishments (Cook, 1913b, p. 335).

Today numerous women serve as military nurses—thanks, in part, to Nightingale's vision of gender diversity and inclusion.

IOM'S VISION

The Committee noted that minority and underprivileged students benefitted from community college ADN programs as the entry level for nursing education and advanced their careers via baccalaureate completion programs. However, the proportion of minority nurses did not represent the diversity of the population. The percentage of diverse nurse faculty members was even lower. Attracting and retaining nursing students and nurses at all levels from racial and ethnic minorities in an issue that must be addressed in nursing education and leadership (IOM, 2011, p. 207). Lack of gender diversity within the profession must also be confronted and resolved to "help offset the shortage of nurses and fill advanced and expanded nursing roles" (IOM, 2011, p. 209).

No formal recommendation was made in *The Future of Nursing* beyond stating that nursing education programs should increase the diversity of their student population (IOM, 2011, p. 207).

Progress toward IOM's Vision

Although the original IOM Report did not establish specific goals to increase diversity in the nursing profession, a pillar in the Campaign for Action is "promoting diversity" (National Academies of Sciences, Engineering, and Medicine, 2016, p. 109). The Campaign's work on diversity is addressed here.

Accomplishments

1. A Campaign-sponsored Diversity Steering Committee of ethnic, racial, and gender minorities advises about diversity measures (National Academies of Sciences, Engineering, and Medicine, 2016, p. 113; Center to Champion Nursing, 2011).

2. The Campaign requires diversity action plans for all states receiving funding from the State Implementation Program (SIP) (National Academies of Sciences, Engineering, and Medicine, 2016, p. 114; Center to Champion Nursing, 2011).

3. The Campaign "sends diversity consultants to states to provide assistance, convenes an Increasing Diversity through Data Learning Collaborative for state Action Coalitions, and compiles resources relating to diversity on the campaign website" (National Academies of Sciences, Engineering, and Medicine, 2016, p. 1115; Center to Champion Nursing, 2011).

4. The Campaign tracks metrics about diversity of RNs, including new graduates and doctoral graduates as well as tracking if states collect race and ethnicity data for their nurses (National Academies of Sciences, Engineering, and Medicine, 2016, p. 1115; Center to Champion nursing, 2011).

Challenges

1. Faculty in baccalaureate master's/doctoral programs are less diverse than students, graduates, and practicing nurses (National Academies of Sciences, Engineering, and Medicine, 2016, p. 125).

2. Funding resources for increasing workforce diversity are not increasing (National Academies of Sciences, Engineering, and Medicine, 2016, p. 125).

3. The Campaign does not have a primary dashboard indicator for diversity because no recommendation or key message was included in *The Future of Nursing* (National Academies of Sciences, Engineering, and Medicine, 2016, p. 115).

4. Hispanic/Latino and African-American nurses are not representative of the population (National Academies of Sciences, Engineering, and Medicine, 2016, p. 129).

5. There is significant variation between nurses and nurse graduates and the diversity of states' populations (National Academies of Sciences, Engineering, and Medicine, 2016, p. 129).

Study Committee's Conclusion

"By making diversity one of its pillars, the Campaign has shone a spotlight on the issue of diversity in the nursing workforce" (National Academies of Sciences, Engineering, and Medicine, 2016, p. 130).

Study Committee's Recommendation

"The Campaign should continue to emphasize recruitment and retention of a diverse nursing workforce as a major priority for both its national efforts and the State Action Coalitions. [The] Campaign should work with others to assess progress and exchange information about strategies that are effective in increasing the diversity of the health workforce" (National Academies of Sciences, Engineering, and Medicine, 2016, p. 130).

Nurses' Vision
Is your healthcare setting on track to meet the IOM recommendation of 80% BSNs by 2020?

1. Yes = 57.14% (116 respondents)

2. No = 42.86% (87 respondents)

Comments

1. "I don't know." (×14)

2. "It is becoming a requirement, but nurses are not being rewarded or compensated to get their BSN. They take on debt for their BSN with nothing in return."

3. "We are a volunteer clinic for the underserved."

4. "We only employ BSNs currently."

5. "Unsure." (×7)

6. "There are a few nursing management/directors that are at the BSN level. There are no incentives at my hospital for obtaining or holding a BSN."

7. "I'm not sure, but it is being talked about in our shared governance meetings."

8. "No idea." (×2)

9. "Unsure, probably not."

10. "Unsure if on track, that is the goal."

11. "Unknown."

12. "I suppose my answer is generationally jaded, but in some ways the diploma and ASN graduates are better

prepared to care for patients. The newer graduates have been steeped in EBP and its importance, but bedside caring and human touch take second to task completion. It is not a wrong move to insist that nurses continually achieve higher education. If BSN is minimum · for practice, then employers should entice and support master's education and organizational certifications. Organizations have to bring back funding for conferences and focus on learning opportunities within their organization."

13. "Yes. They (BSNs) do function at a higher level, and research shows that they do. BSNs have been introduced to the concepts of EBP and research in their programs whereas ADNs and LVNs have not really had the opportunity to learn about them."

14. "No. Not enough BSN nurses applying & RNs are not being required to return for their BSN. There is no structure for an increased wage for BSN RNs. The job description does not indicate a performance difference."

Does your healthcare setting make diversity a priority in workforce hiring and retention?

1. Yes = 64.57% (144 respondents)

2. No = 35.43% (79 respondents)

Comments

1. "Support for Indian Nurse Society, giving a diversity award to nurses for learning and caring for another cultural group."

2. "Our community is diversity rich!! But we need to move from just people of color, to a dialogue that includes conversations about religious and sexual

diversity. For the first time in reporting history, working single females outnumber married women. Empowering single staff is also a demographic that needs to be looked at and supported. Also different dietary lifestyles. We have 10,000 staff members, but as the largest health system, can't we support environmental issues and use that leverage for positive change?"

3. "Unsure." (×4)

4. "This does not seem to be a priority. We rely on contract labor/travel nurses."

5. "I teach full time and work as a volunteer in a primary care clinic once per week. Both sites highly value diversity."

6. "I don't know." (×2)

7. "Shortage of nurses at my healthcare setting—feel that they just hire anyone with BSN."

8. "The institution doesn't require BSN to hire for that reason—doesn't require RN-to-BSN either."

9. "Yes, almost to the point of alienating the rest of the staff."

10. "They hire on nursing merits, not skin color."

11. "No idea."

12. "We do not have diverse applicants in our local area. We would support a diverse workforce, but other than gender, we do not have a sufficient applicant pool."

CHAPTER 6

Double the Number of Nurses with Doctorates by 2020 (2010)

"So shall we do everything in our power to become proficient, not only in knowing the symptoms and what is to be done, but in knowing the 'Reason Why' of such symptoms, and *why* such and such a thing is done; and so on, till we can someday TRAIN OTHERS *to know the 'reason why.'*"

—F. Nightingale
(Nightingale, 2012, p. 70)

Florence Nightingale's vision of trained nurses was an antecedent of today's focus on advanced degrees. She dedicated a portion of the Nightingale Fund for training of nurse midwives and collaborated with the staff of King's College Hospital and the Sisters of St. John's House to develop this advanced role in England. Most European countries had a government-sponsored school for midwives. The school at King's College Hospital was the first one in England and was only possible with Nightingale's intervention. Women were selected by parishes in the countryside and completed a six-month course before returning to their communities to practice midwifery among poor women who wouldn't otherwise have care during childbirth. The Head Nurse was an experienced midwife, who acted as a resource for the students during their training period. Obstetricians taught the students to care for women during labor and delivery, and students delivered babies in homes as outpatients during their experience at King's College Hospital. The hospital was poor, and Nightingale had to create a maternity department as a new service as well as funding for room and board for the student midwives. The success of this practice initiative resulted in additional midwifery training at St. Thomas' Hospital (Cook, 1913a). Nightingale considered midwifery a career for educated women and wrote a book in 1871 called *Introductory Notes on Lying-in Institutions* that described an ideal school for training midwives and called public attention to the importance of cleanliness to reduce mortality in maternity wards to levels commensurate with home deliveries (Cook, 1913b, pp. 196–197). Her influence increased the number and prestige of trained midwives for the benefit of poor women in England.

"Schools of nursing, with support from private and public funders, academic administrators and university trustees, and accrediting bodies, should double the number of nurses with a doctorate by 2020 to add to the cadre of nurse faculty and researchers, with attention to increasing diversity" (IOM, 2011, p. 13).

The complexity of future health care will require nurses with advanced degrees as APRNs, nurse researchers, and nurse faculty. As previously stated, APRNs' role in care of underserved patient populations in primary care and community settings requires minimally a master's degree in nursing accompanied by applicable certification (IOM, 2011, p. 196). Many nurse faculty members are also master's prepared nurses. There are two doctoral degrees: the Doctor of Nursing Practice (DNP) and the PhD. Nurses with PhDs conduct research that advances practice and may be employed as university faculty or leaders in health care systems and academic sites (IOM, 2011, p. 194).

The DNP is a newer nursing role where the nurse is employed as a leader in clinical practice. This degree complements other practice degrees, such as PharmD. and MD. Nurses with DNPs use clinical research evidence to improve systems of care and organization performance (IOM, 2011, p. 194). The Committee did not address the effect of this role "on patient outcomes, costs, quality of care, and access in clinical settings" (IOM, 2011, p. 195) because of insufficient evidence about improved outcomes when the IOM report was initially developed. At that time, only 13% of registered nurses had attained a graduate-level degree, and less than 1% held a doctoral degree in nursing or a nursing-related discipline (IOM, 2011, p. 195).

PhD programs have not grown as the need for their skills in research and education has expanded. The Committee cited three reasons for this gap:

1. The number of nurses with advanced degrees is inadequate (IOM, 2011, p. 195).

2. The benefits and salaries for faculty members are insufficient for nurses with advanced degrees compared to employment in clinical facilities (IOM, 2011, p. 196).

3. The nursing culture advocates obtaining clinical expertise before entering graduate education (IOM, 2011, p. 196).

APRNs seek certification to validate their skills and knowledge. Certification must be renewed at specific intervals and includes requirements for practice hours and requirements for continuing education in the practice specialty. Complexity in health care will require additional competencies in multiple functions. Coursework and clinical requirements in advanced practice programs must reflect role transitions in the future health care environment. The Committee did not distinguish between nurses with master's degrees and DNP degrees in its report (IOM, 2011, p. 197).

PhD-prepared nurses are too few to address critical research in nursing education and the growth of nursing science. Both are essential to achieve outcomes that improve patient-focused care by expert clinicians (IOM, 2011, p. 198). The Committee realized that "nursing's research capacity has been largely overlooked in the development of strategies for responding to the shortage of nurses or effecting the necessary transformation of the nursing profession" (IOM, 2011, p. 199).

To address these issues, the Committee recommended the following approaches:

1. Monitoring of each accredited school of nursing by the NLN Accrediting Commission and the Commission on Collegiate Nursing Education "to ensure that at least 10 percent of all baccalaureate graduates matriculate into a master's or doctoral program within 5 years of graduation" (IOM, 2011, p. 13).

2. HRSA, the Department of Labor, and public and private funders "should expand funding for programs offering accelerated graduate degrees for nurses to

increase the production of master's and doctoral nurse graduates and to increase the diversity of nurse faculty, scientists, and researchers" (IOM, 2011, p. 13).

3. Creation by trustees and administrators of colleges and universities of "salary and benefit packages that are market competitive to recruit and retain highly quali- fied academic and clinical nurse faculty" (IOM, 2011, p. 13).

How has the supply of qualified nurses with doctorates fared since the 2010 IOM recommendations? The next section addresses the status of nurses with doctorates in the years since the publication of the IOM Report.

Promote Nurses' Pursuit of Doctoral Degrees (2015)

"Ought they not to look upon themselves as future leaders—as those who will have to train others?"
—F. Nightingale (Nightingale, 2012, p. 69)

NIGHTINGALE'S VISION

Florence Nightingale realized that formal nursing education had to advance, not remain in stasis. The Nightingale School was a positive start, and she promoted nurses' pursuit of "obtaining a practical and scientific training, and of raising by degrees the standard of education and character among nurses as a class. From year to year the other hospitals were assisted from the mother school with trained superin- tendents and staff and new centres were formed with the same objects, and it may well be said that the seed thus sown by Miss Nightingale through the means of the Fund has been mainly instrumental in raising the calling of nurses to the position it now holds" (Cook, 1913a, p. 465). This statement was made by the Council of the Nightingale Fund in 1910, and nursing education followed Nightingale's pattern in numerous countries worldwide. Her high stan- dards promoted nurses' attainment of additional knowledge, resulting in revisions to nursing curriculums. Although she was actively involved in major initiatives affecting the health of people throughout the world, Nightingale never lost track of the progress of the school and the importance of excellence in education and practice. While she was examining Indian sanitation issues, she also revised the curriculum of the Nightingale School so probationers attended the National Training School of Cookery to enhance their understanding of patients' nutritional issues (Cook, 1913b, p. 326). In this and other instances, Nightingale promoted nurses' pursuit of knowledge to enhance their practice in all settings.

Progress toward IOM's Vision

The Study Committee reviewed progress toward doubling the number of doctoral-prepared registered nurses by 2020 as well as how graduates are employed in academic and health care settings.

Accomplishments

1. Private foundations, the American Cancer Society, and the BlueCross Blue Shield CareFirst Project RN have provided funding for nurses to attend graduate programs to attain DNPs and PhDs since the publication of *The Future of Nursing* (National Academies of Sciences, Engineering, and Medicine, 2016, pp. 85–87).

2. Enrollment in doctoral programs has risen since the IOM report. DNP enrollment has more than doubled, and PhD enrollment has grown by 15% (National Academies of Sciences, Engineering, and Medicine, 2016, p. 87).

3. There are significantly more DNP programs (from 20 in 2006 to 262 in 2014) and slightly more PhD programs (from 103 in 2006 to 133 in 2014) (National Academies of Sciences, Engineering, and Medicine, 2016, p. 87).

4. Growth has occurred in baccalaureate-to-DNP and master's-to-DNP programs (National Academies of Sciences, Engineering, and Medicine, 2016, p. 88).

Challenges

1. Doubling the number of nurses with doctorates is insufficient to address faculty and research needs (National Academies of Sciences, Engineering, and Medicine, 2016, p. 90).

2. There is confusion about the role of the DNP "with regard to research and knowledge generation, leadership, and advanced practice" (National Academies of Sciences, Engineering, and Medicine, 2016, p. 90).

3. Many schools cannot admit qualified applicants without additional faculty due to "insufficient funds, unwillingness to commit to hiring full-time employees, noncompetitive salaries, an inability to recruit qualified individuals or those with the right specialties or research or teaching interests, the limited number of doctorally prepared nurses, and a lack of qualified applicants in the school's area" (National Academies of Sciences, Engineering, and Medicine, 2016, p. 91).

4. Nurse faculty are aging, and significant turnover is expected from faculty retirements (National Academies of Sciences, Engineering, and Medicine, 2016, p. 91).

Study Committee's Conclusion

"The recommendation of *The Future of Nursing* calling for a doubling of the number of nurses with a doctorate by 2020 is not specific about growth in particular types of doctoral programs (DNP, PhD in nursing, PhD in another field)" (National Academies of Sciences, Engineering, and Medicine, 2016, p. 91).

Study Committee's Recommendation

"As nurses are increasingly looked to for leadership in health care, advanced education in clinical care, research, education, and other areas (including public policy and business), advanced degrees will be more useful than ever. Information exists and is readily available about the number of nurses with higher degrees in the workforce. However, the breakdown of nurses with these degrees (particularly those with non-nursing advanced degrees), the settings in which they practice, and the types of work they do is less accessible. Additional efforts are needed to clarify the roles of PhD and DNP nurses, especially with regard to teaching and research" (National Academies of Sciences, Engineering, and Medicine, 2016, p. 92).

Nurses' Vision

Another recommendation is to double the number of nurses with doctorates by 2020. Do you or other RNs in your healthcare setting have a doctoral degree (PhD, DNP)?

1. Yes = 36.89% (83 respondents)

2. No = 63.11% (142 respondents)

Comments

1. "I don't know a single RN with a doctorate. I've asked around about higher education, and the consensus is that because the hospital doesn't employ NPs or give a pay raise for having a MSN, there is no reason for it."

2. "Two nurses are completing their PhDs. The organization does not off-load work in order to support the time needed to achieve the degree. There are minimal tuition reimbursement programs."

3. "I have not looked at the clinical ladder to see how nurses are supported to achieve doctorates. But for a new nurse looking to move up, there are few open options in this current healthcare model."

4. "Not much support financially. DNPs are either CNOs, or assistant CNOs, and PhDs are primarily nurse scientists. Nurses burn out and then start looking for academic jobs, so they pursue a DNP or PhD."

5. "Currently in DNP program."

6. "Not sure." (×2)

7. "But MPhil in nursing."

8. "RNs in leadership have DNP."

9. "I don't, but leadership and various other RNs do."

10. "Maybe 1 or 2."

11. "Unknown."

12. "Several master's, mostly BSN."

13. "I am almost done with my DNP."

14. "There is a loan repayment program here, but HR has stated several times that it will not be approved for degrees not necessary for one's job function."

CHAPTER 7

Ensure that Nurses Engage in Lifelong Learning (2010)

"We do not calculate the future by our experience of the past. What right have we to expect that, if we have not improved during the last six months, we shall during the next six?"

—F. Nightingale
(Nightingale, 2012, p. 50)

NIGHTINGALE'S VISION

Florence Nightingale was an avowed proponent of lifelong learning for herself as well as other nurses. Her position enabled her to role model this behavior throughout her life. Her love of knowledge began as a child when she and her sister were home-schooled by their father. She studied geography, languages, and mathematics. As a teenager, she read classical works in Latin and Greek. When her father gave the girls homework, Nightingale often awoke at 4 a.m. to study and prepare for the day's lesson. She learned to write essays that later prepared her for significant contributions to literature and science. Her education was supplemented by trips abroad to France and Italy, where she was exposed to society, politics, and a passion for statistics that she enjoyed for the rest of her life. Her diary included all these topics as well as references to art and notes about architecture (Cook, 1913a).

When she traveled, Nightingale immersed herself in books and this continued when her family visited Egypt and Greece. In Egypt, she studied the life of religious sisterhoods in health care and education. In Greece, she admired the beauty of the country and political discourse there. When Nightingale became a young woman, she spent time studying hospital and nursing organizations in France and Germany. She would use this knowledge throughout her career and learned from experts in many fields as she pursued reform in years to come. These experts included statisticians, architects, sanitarians, and nutritionists (Cook, 1913a).

Nightingale continued her pursuit of learning after her return from the Crimea. She visited numerous military and public hospitals for many years to develop her expertise on hospital construction and management. Her skills as a statistician were enhanced when she read Adolphe Quetelet's meteorological studies. Quetelet was a statistician and Nightingale was intrigued by an essay in which he "showed the possibility of applying the statistical method to social dynamics, and deduced from such method various conclusions with regard to the physical and intellectual qualities of man" (Cook, 1913a, p. 429).

Nightingale devoured facts and figures, but she also enjoyed discussions about philosophy and religion. Most of all, she never stopped learning and sharing her knowledge with an audience around the world. She was a remarkable role model to nurses and others for engaging in lifelong learning.

IOM'S VISION

"Accrediting bodies, schools of nursing, health care organizations, and continuing competency educators from multiple health professions should collaborate to ensure that nurses and nursing students and faculty continue their education and engage in lifelong learning to gain the competencies needed to provide care for diverse populations across the lifespan" (IOM, 2011, p. 13).

As health care changes and becomes more complex, graduation from a nursing program and licensure will not ensure competent and safe provision of care in multiple locations from acute care to community and transitional settings throughout a nurse's career. Traditional competencies—"care management and coordination, patient education, public health intervention, and transitional care" (IOM, 2011, p. 199)—will continue to exist, but must be aligned with new competencies—"decision making, quality improvement, systems thinking, and team leadership" (IOM, 2011, p. 2. 199)—for nursing students and nurses at all academic levels. Competency-based nursing education must be connected to expectations for clinical performance. Nursing core competencies are beyond simple task performance. These competencies overlap and serve as "a foundation for decision-making skills under a variety of clinical situations across all care settings" (IOM, 2011, p. 200).

The Committee decided that educational content must be redesigned beyond adding content to current nursing programs to adequately teach all evolving competencies. They believed that establishing a common set of core competencies would improve communication and collaboration across disciplines. The Committee also endorsed a uniform set of nursing core competencies to inform standards within nursing education programs. Definition of core competencies would involve partnership between "nurse educators, professional organizations, and health care organizations and providers" (IOM, 2011, p. 201).

The Committee advocated for competency-based assessment in both nursing education and nursing performance. Competency attainment in coursework expects students to validate their understanding and performance of the competency. Competency attainment in performance expects the nurse to understand the theory behind the competency and apply it in practice (IOM, 2011, pp. 201–202). This competence must continue throughout the nurse's career. After completion of formal education, continuing education has been the venue to acquire and maintain emerging competencies.

Continuing education programs are not always based on evidence, and a clear link may not be present between the program and required competency. The Committee supported engagement of all health disciplines in team learning to improve population health and patient-focused care. Achieving this vision involves increasing nurses' capacity for lifelong learning through "both continuing competence and advanced degrees" (IOM, 2011, p. 202).

Supporting recommendations by the Committee included the following:

1. Partnership between faculty and health care organizations "to develop and prioritize competencies so curricula can be updated regularly" (IOM, 2011, p. 13)

2. Requirement for all nursing students to "demonstrate a comprehensive set of clinical performance competencies that encompass the knowledge and skills needed to provide care across settings and the lifespan" (IOM, 2011, p. 14)

3. Requirement for all faculty members "to participate in continuing professional development and to perform with cutting-edge competence in practice, teaching, and research" (IOM, 2011, p. 14)

4. Support by nursing schools and health care organizations to "foster a culture of lifelong learning and provide resources for interprofessional continuing competency programs" (IOM, 2011, p. 14)

5. Regular evaluation and updates by organizations offering competency programs "for adaptability, flexibility, accessibility, and impact on clinical outcomes" (IOM, 2011, p. 14).

What progress has been made on these recommendations since the original IOM report? That is examined in the following section.

Promote Nurses' Interprofessional and Lifelong Learning (2015)

"And to nurse . . . is a field, a road, of which one may safely say: There is no end—no end in what we may be learning every day. There is a well-known Society abroad (for charitable works) of which the Members go through two years' probation on their first entering, but after ten years they return and go through a second probation of one year. This is one of the most striking recognitions I know of the fact that progress is always to be made: that grown-up people, even of middle-age, ought always to have their education going on. But only those *can* learn *after* middle age who have gone on learning up to middle age."
—F. Nightingale (Nightingale, 2012, pp. 3–4)

Many of Nightingale's addresses to her probationers promoted lifelong learning. She realized that a one-year training program would not be enough for proficient practice. Nursing and healthcare were advancing, and a limited knowledge base wouldn't benefit patients or the nurses themselves. In her own words, "For us who nurse, our nursing is a thing in which, unless we are making *progress* every year, every month, every week—take my word for it, we are going *back*. The more experience we gain, the more progress we can make. The progress you make in your year's training with us is as nothing to what you must make every year *after* your year's training is over. A woman who thinks in herself: 'Now I am a full Nurse, a skilled Nurse, I have learnt all that there is to be learnt'—take my word for it, she does not know what a Nurse is, and she never will know; she is gone back already" (Cook, 1913b, p. 264).

Nightingale was also concerned about interprofessional relationships between nurses and physicians. She had experienced both support and antagonism from surgeons during her work in the Crimea and knew that patients benefitted when both disciplines worked together. She also understood that education for nurses did make a positive difference in interprofessional learning and collaboration. As she aptly remarked, "My principle has always been: that we should give the best training we could to any woman of any class, of any sect, paid or unpaid, who had the requisite qualifications, moral, intellectual, and physical, for the vocation of a Nurse. Unquestionably, the educated will be more likely to rise to the post of Superintendents, *not* because they are ladies, *but* because they are educated. The relation of a nursing staff to the medical officers is that of the building staff to an architect. And neither can know its business if not trained to it. To pit the medical school against the nurse-training school is to pit the hour-hand against the minute-hand" (Cook, 1913b, p. 270).

Progress toward IOM's Vision

The Study Committee reviewed the progress toward continuing competence and lifelong learning since publication of *The Future of Nursing*.

Accomplishments

1. Joint Accreditation for Interprofessional Education has streamlined the accreditation process and established standards through joint collaboration by the ANCC (nursing), ACCME (medicine), and ACPE (pharmacy) (National Academies of Sciences, Engineering, and Medicine, 2016, p. 93).

2. Three states (Washington, Georgia, and Oklahoma) have implemented "continuing competency requirements for nurses" (National Academies of Sciences, Engineering, and Medicine, 2016, p. 92).

Challenges

1. There is no dashboard indicator for the Campaign to evaluate progress toward continuing competence and lifelong learning (National Academies of Sciences, Engineering, and Medicine, 2016, p. 92).

2. Continuing education has not met the needs of the "increasingly complex, team-based health care system" (National Academies of Sciences, Engineering, and Medicine, 2016, p. 95).

3. There is no single complete data source about continuing education for nurses and lifelong learning (National Academies of Sciences, Engineering, and Medicine, 2016, p. 95).

4. There is a lack of evidence if "nurse certification and credentialing lead to better patient outcomes" (National Academies of Sciences, Engineering, and Medicine, 2016, p. 92).

5. Cost of certification and inadequate organizational support for its value remain barriers to attainment and maintenance by nurses (National Academies of Sciences, Engineering, and Medicine, 2016, p. 96).

6. Education of nurses as health professionals is still focused on acute care rather than other health care settings (National Academies of Sciences, Engineering, and Medicine, 2016, p. 96).

Study Committee's Conclusion

"The current health care context makes interprofessional continuing education more important than ever. Current efforts by health care delivery organizations, accreditors, and state regulatory boards to promote these programs need to be expanded and promoted" (National Academies of Sciences, Engineering, and Medicine, 2016, p. 97).

Study Committee's Recommendation

"The Campaign should encourage nursing organizations, education programs, and professional societies, as well as individual nurses, to make lifelong learning a priority so that nurses are prepared to work in evolving health care environments. Lifelong learning should include continuing education that will enable nurses to gain, preserve, and measure the skills needed in the variety of environments and settings in which health care will be provided going forward, particularly community-based, outpatient, long-term care, primary care, and ambulatory settings. Nurses should work with other health care professionals to create opportunities for interprofessional collaboration and education. The Campaign could serve as a convener to bring together stakeholders from multiple areas of health care to discuss opportunities and strategies for interdisciplinary collaboration in this area" (National Academies of Sciences, Engineering, and Medicine, 2016, p. 98).

Nurses' Vision

Does your healthcare setting support lifelong learning as a priority for nurses?

Yes = 74.24% (170 respondents)

No = 25.76% (59 respondents)

Comments

1. "We use a Fellowship program that lasts a year in order to help bedside BSNs to learn EBP well. They many times decide that they will return to school for a MSN after finding out they can create a great EBP project."

2. "Collaborative care teams have nurses from different levels interacting for common goals. I see recent grads struggling with wanting certification, but unsure of financial burdens. They are newlyweds and have student loans to pay. Many have young children. My organization asks that you pursue education in addition to working hours. Many already work a lot of overtime."

3. "Unsure."

4. "Sharing CE programs and collaborating on continuing education programs, particularly for night staff.
   Being an example to be open minded and continue to
   ask questions, discuss unique patient care situations."

5. "The clinic I work in has weekly interprofessional
   education sessions."

6. "In theory."

7. "No money for continuing education even for required
   certification unless full-time."

CHAPTER 8

Prepare and Enable Nurses to Lead Change to Advance Health (2010)

"As we find in all history and true fable that the meanest causes universally multiplied produce the greatest effects, let us not think it other than a fitting sacrifice to the Eternal and Perfect One to look into the lowest habits of great peoples, in order, if we may, to awaken them to a sense of the injury they are doing themselves and the good they might do themselves. Much of the willingness for education is due to the fact, appreciated by them, that education makes money. But would not the same appreciation,

if enlightened, show them that loss
of health, loss of strength, loss of life,
is loss of money, the greatest loss of
money we know? And we may truly
say that every sanitary improvement
which saves health and life is worth
its weight in gold."

—F. Nightingale, Address to the
Peoples of India (Cook, 1913b, p. 179)

NIGHTINGALE'S VISION

Florence Nightingale's Crimean experiences provided her with an insight that she used to prepare and enable nurses to lead change to advance health. When she arrived at the Barrack Hospital in Scutari, Nightingale observed that patient care was delegated to untrained orderlies. Many of these men were negligent in performing their duties. Because the number of nurses was limited, the work of these orderlies was essential. She began instructing them in their duties, including the importance of proper sanitation and hand washing. As her influence with the orderlies grew, sanitation reforms occurred (Cook, 1913a, p. 219).

Nightingale's correspondence with the Secretary at War, Sidney Herbert, about the poor condition of the hospital and reforms needed to improve them also included her observation of the orderlies. She described "the total inefficiency of the Hospital Or-

derly System as it now is. The French have a permanent system of Orderlies trained for the purpose, who do not re-enter the ranks. It is too late for us to organize this. But if the convalescents, being good Orderlies, were not sent away to the Crimea as soon as they have learnt their work—if the Commander-in-Chief would call upon the Commanding Officer of each Regiment to select ten men from each as Hospital Orderlies to form a depot here (not young soldiers, but men of good character), this would give some hope of organizing an efficient corps" (Cook, 1913a, p. 225). She also expressed concern for the health of the orderlies who also experienced significant illness and mortality.

Nightingale recommended, "The Orderlies ought to be well paid, well fed, well-housed. They are now overworked, ill fed, and underpaid" (Cook, 1913a, p. 226).

Under the supervision and training of Nightingale and her nurses, the orderlies gained proficiency in the tasks assigned to them. This change in performing their duties advanced the health of the soldiers by greater attention to their needs and the hospital environment. In later years, Nightingale worked to reform the Army Medical Corps, and the presence of female nurses confirmed her vision that "the most important function of the female nurse was the education of the male orderly" (Cook, 1913b, p. 342). When one of her nurses went to Suez during the Egyptian Campaign in 1885, Nightingale's advice encouraged her to continue to train the orderlies to care for soldiers in battlefield hospitals. Her counsel prepared and enabled this nurse and others to lead change that advanced soldiers' health by attention to the orderlies (Cook, 1913b).

IOM'S VISION

"Nurses, nursing education programs, and nursing associations should prepare the nursing workforce to assume leadership positions across all levels, while public, private, and governmental health care decision makers should ensure that leadership positions are available to, and filled by nurses" (IOM, 2011, p. 14).

The IOM Committee considered all nurses as leaders and realized that a new set of leadership skills and competencies would be required for nurses to lead change and advance health in a changing environment. Collaboration in interprofessional teams is a worthy aim, but it is not easy to achieve in practice. Every nurse must be prepared to lead in locations from acute care to community and home health care settings by advocating for their patients and families (IOM, 2011, pp. 227–228).

Basic leadership skills must be taught in nursing education programs, and faculty must prepare students for their future careers. Students should be encouraged to begin leading in local nonprofit organizations and within the National Student Nurses Association (NSNA) to develop their skills in interacting with other health care disciplines and the public (IOM, 2011, pp. 229–231).

Staff nurses have an opportunity "to design new models of care to improve quality, efficiency, and safety" (IOM, 2011, p. 234). To be successful, this will require mutual accountability by the health care team as well as "communication, conflict resolution, and negotiating skills necessary to succeed in leadership and partnership roles" (IOM, 2011, p. 234). Community health nurses are change agents in promoting health and safety by responding to communicable diseases and other health risks. They must play a leadership role in collaborating with "community, state, and federal officials to assure the health and safety of the public" (IOM, 2011, p. 235). Chief nursing officers (CNOs) must participate in the highest levels of decision making about patient care. However, they are confronted with changes in reporting relationships that reduce their clout and significant increases in responsibilities that infringe on their time to contribute to key decisions (IOM, 2011, p. 235). Nurses are also "underrepresented on institution and hospital boards, either their own or others" (IOM, 2011, p. 236). Such boards now focus on quality and safety in addition to business practices and financial considerations.

Nurse board members can significantly influence safety and quality improvement issues. CNOs must prepare for and seek opportunities to serve on boards of health organizations and encourage their staff leaders to serve on important boards and committees in the organization and in the community (IOM, 2011, p. 238). Nurse researchers' leadership role focuses on creating "new models of quality care that are evidence-based, patient-centered, affordable, and accessible to diverse populations" (IOM, 2011, p. 238). Nursing organizations must find common ground "to offer evidence-based solutions for improvements in patient care" (IOM, 2011, pp. 239–240).

The Committee believed that three approaches are essential for nurses to undertake leadership roles in advancing health. These approaches include "leadership programs for nurses; mentorship; and involvement in the policy-making process, including political engagement" (IOM, 2011, p. 241). Various leadership programs exist that include formal training and education, and several nursing organizations have mentorship programs for their members. Many nurses have served in government and legislative offices to increase their leadership involvement in policy decisions. Focusing on improving the quality of patient care while reducing costs is an area that nurses excel in and can be achieved with political engagement when nurses (1) develop alliances in their professional community, (2) align with key policy makers, and (3) locate allies outside nursing to promote common goals (IOM, 2011, p. 250).

These perspectives about preparing and enabling nurses as leaders to advance health were identified by the Committee during its work. Supporting recommendations included the following:

1. Nurses must continue their education and use leadership skills to assume responsibility for "their personal and professional growth" (IOM, 2011, p. 14).

2. Nursing associations and societies "should provide leadership development, mentoring programs, and opportunities to lead for all their members" (IOM, 2011, p. 14).

3. Business practices and leadership theory should be integrated in nursing education programs "across the curriculum, including clinical practice" (IOM, 2011, p. 14).

4. Health care decision makers at all levels should incorporate nursing representatives "on boards, on executive management teams, and in other key leadership positions" (IOM, 2011, p. 14).

The next section discusses progress in the first five years and the challenges affecting the leadership of nurses in care delivery redesign and health care payment systems.

Promote Nurses' Involvement in Redesign of Care Delivery and Payment Systems (2015)

"Let each Founder train as many in his or her spirit as he or she can. Then the pupils will in their turn be Founders also." —F. Nightingale (Cook, 1913b, p. 246)

"Miss Nightingale's scheme for Uniform Hospital Statistics seems to require for its realization a more diffused passion for statistics and a greater delicacy of statistical conscience than a voluntary and competitive system of hospitals is likely to create." —E. T. Cook (Cook, 1913a, p. 434)

NIGHTINGALE'S VISION

Throughout her career, Nightingale was a passionate statistician. Redesigning payment systems required in-depth statistical analysis to persuade political leaders about the need for change. Unfortunately, many of these leaders lacked knowledge of how statistical analysis could improve health care. Her time in Scutari showed Florence Nightingale the inadequacy of Army statistics on mortality and the need for Army reform. Money in the treasury was not always available for reforms to improve soldiers' health. Nightingale converted her statistics into diagrams showing preventable deaths during the Crimean War and soldiers' mortality at home. She widely distributed these diagrams to galvanize administrative and public support for reforms. Her collaboration with the Chairman of the Royal Commission on the sanitary condition of the British Army resulted in funding for barracks and hospital construction to improve soldiers' health that was unanimously approved by the House of Commons. Her persistence resulted in safer housing and improved nutrition for soldiers, resulting in reduction of mortality and morbidity in the Army (Cook, 1913a).

Progress toward IOM's Vision

In *The Future of Nursing*, the IOM Committee defined no metric to track whether nurses were being prepared to lead and leading change to advance health. The IOM Report's recommendations concentrated on how the nursing profession can prepare itself for leadership roles (National Academies of Sciences, Engineering, and Medicine, 2016, p. 148).

Accomplishments

1. Some nursing programs have integrated leadership and entrepreneurship into their programs or by combining these classes with another school (National Academies of Sciences, Engineering, and Medicine, 2016, p. 146).

2. Nursing associations and societies are actively sponsoring entrepreneurial and leadership programs for nurses (National Academies of Sciences, Engineering, and Medicine, 2016, p. 146).

3. Philanthropic and private organizations have supported programs to train and educate nurses in leadership skills (National Academies of Sciences, Engineering, and Medicine, 2016, p. 147).

4. The Campaign's "leveraging nursing leadership" pillar stresses preparation of nurses for leadership and advancing nurses as leaders in health care (National Academies of Sciences, Engineering, and Medicine, 2016, p. 148).

5. The Campaign has created the "Breakthrough Leadership in Nursing Awards program to recognize and advance 10 nurse leaders" (National Academies of Sciences, Engineering, and Medicine, 2016, p. 148).

6. More nurses have been appointed to private health-related boards (National Academies of Sciences, Engineering, and Medicine, 2016, p. 151).

Challenges

1. No one source exists "about nurse training in leadership, entrepreneurship, or innovation" (National Academies of Sciences, Engineering, and Medicine, 2016, p. 148).

2. Data about nurses serving as leaders to advance health is "fragmented and incomplete" (National Academies of Sciences, Engineering, and Medicine, 2016, p. 151).

3. More emphasis must occur for nurses to serve on hospital boards (National Academies of Sciences, Engineering, and Medicine, 2016, p. 149).

Study Committee's Conclusion

"To assess progress on leadership development, it is necessary to track programs and courses in leadership, entrepreneurship, and management in which nurses are participating" (National Academies of Sciences, Engineering, and Medicine, 2016, p. 149).

"More focus is needed on nurses serving in leadership positions other than on private boards" (National Academies of Sciences, Engineering, and Medicine, 2016, p. 151).

Study Committee's Recommendation

"The Campaign should work with payers, health care organizations, providers, employers, and regulators to involve nurses in the redesign of care delivery and payment systems. To this end, the Campaign should encourage nurses to serve in executive and leadership positions in government, for-profit, and nonprofit organizations; health care delivery systems (e.g., as hospital chief executive officers or chief operations officers); and advisory committees (National Academies of Sciences, Engineering, and Medicine, 2016, p. 156).

Communicate with Wider and More Diverse Audience to Gain Broad Support for Campaign (2015)

"Statisticians, sanitary engineers, architects, and other experts were all in correspondence with Miss Nightingale during the preparation of her Report (on the health of the Army). In every branch of her inquiry she was equally thorough; consulting the best authorities, collecting the essential facts." —E. T. Cook (Cook, 1913a, p. 352)

NIGHTINGALE'S VISION

Nightingale's diverse reform efforts required a diverse team to accomplish her goals. She had an uncanny ability to collaborate with the right individuals and groups on various issues. Early in her nursing career, Nightingale became the first civilian nurse to command nurses in a war zone. After landing in Scutari, she was shocked at the condition of the hospital there: inadequate supplies and equipment, poor sanitation, lack of nourishing food for patients, and a squalid environment. She and her nurses could clean the floors with scrub brushes, but that was only a starting point to improving conditions for the wounded soldiers housed there. Nightingale recognized that a diverse team was essential to effect positive changes. She began by employing soldiers' wives to wash linens—shirts and bedding—in

hot water. She found a location in a Turkish house and collaborated with the Engineer's Office to install boilers. In addition to using some of her own funds, Nightingale used some the funds dedicated to her by the *Times*. The press was her ally and informed the British public, royalty, and government of her activities, challenges, and successes. Her next step in her campaign to improve the care of these soldiers involved the inadequacy of their food. There was one kitchen at one end of the Barrack that had to serve all patients who were housed in an area three to four miles long. Serving dinner took up to four hours and was inedible for men at the end of the line. Within 10 days, Nightingale opened two more kitchens in different locations and had three supplementary boilers repaired to prepare starches (Cook, 1913a).

When the British Ambassador told the Commissioner of the *Times* Fund that nothing was needed in Scutari's hospitals and suggested funds be used to build a church, Nightingale spoke with the Commissioner and opened a store instead to supply clothing, kettles and pans, food for special diets, and utensils. She used this store to fill requisitions by surgeons for their patients, and women volunteers handled the distribution of supplies. The purveyor who was responsible for supplies in the war zone couldn't meet the surgeons' requests because he refused to release them without action by the Board of Survey, and the wheels of bureaucracy moved slowly. Nightingale had no such constraints and brought in supplies that the purveyor didn't or wouldn't stock. The *Times* reporter was also resourceful in obtaining funding for the store's inventory (Cook, 1913a).

The next issue in her campaign for the soldiers involved restoring unsafe wards to accommodate 800 more patients. Nightingale collaborated with a senior medical officer at the hospital and described the urgency of this request to the Ambassador's wife, who was his liaison to the hospital leaders. The chief of the engineers started the work, but all 125 workmen went on strike. Nightingale contracted 200 other workers, and the project was rapidly completed. Two weeks later, 500 men occupied beds in these updated wards (Cook, 1913a).

Nightingale demonstrated in multiple instances during her service in Scutari and the Crimea an ability to collaborate and communicate with diverse groups and individuals. She gained their support for her successful campaign to provide the care soldier patients deserved.

IOM'S VISION

"Nurses should be full partners with physicians and other health professionals, in redesigning health care in the United States" (IOM, 2011, p. 221).

For nurses to effectively lead change to advance health, they must align themselves with multiple stakeholders, within and outside health care. The Committee asked nurses to collaborate with new colleagues "from business, government, and philanthropy to state and national medical associations to consumer groups" (IOM, 2011, p. 251). Nurses' personal and professional relationships can lead to their success as leaders in care delivery and research. Although interprofessional collaboration in teams will guide change in health care, nurses must also develop relationships with other community stakeholders to become full partners in "quality improvement, care coordination, and health promotion" (IOM, 2011, p. 251). Such alliances will ensure that nurses are "at the table" when decisions are made. The Committee promoted nurses' representation "on the boards of private nonprofit and philanthropic organizations, which do not provide health care services, but often have a large impact on health care decisions" (IOM, 2011, p. 251). Some of these organizations have physicians, but not nurses, on their boards. Although the Committee advised nurses to collaborate in diverse settings by employing leadership competencies, no recommendation was made about strategies to gain additional allies within and outside health care (IOM, 2011).

Progress toward IOM's Vision

Although the Committee set no goal for nurses to engage additional stakeholders, the Campaign recognized the importance of a broad alliance to gain support for nurses to lead change and advance health. They developed communication strategies to support State Action Coalitions' involvement with diverse stakeholders who shared common beliefs.

Accomplishments

1. Action Coalitions with staff assigned to communications have demonstrated success in communicating with other stakeholders about their activities (National Academies of Sciences, Engineering, and Medicine, 2016, p. 151).

2. The Campaign used strategic means of communication to connect with "nursing and higher education

committees" (National Academies of Sciences, Engineering, and Medicine, 2016, p. 152).

3. Campaign leaders and representatives have spoken at seminars and conferences throughout the United States "to raise awareness of and inform key audiences about the recommendations of *The Future of Nursing*, and to gather relevant data and information to advance Campaign goals" (National Academies of Sciences, Engineering, and Medicine, 2016, p. 152).

4. Campaign volunteers can access online materials "to use in engaging media, policy makers, and interested stakeholders" (National Academies of Sciences, Engineering, and Medicine, 2016, p. 152).

Challenges

1. The Campaign must move beyond engaging nurses to involve additional outside stakeholders (National Academies of Sciences, Engineering, and Medicine, 2016, p. 152).

2. Most Action Coalitions have tried to connect with diverse stakeholders but need more non-nursing representatives to advance their goals (National Academies of Sciences, Engineering, and Medicine, 2016, p. 152).

3. The Campaign must expand its communication strategies to attract a broader and diverse audience (National Academies of Sciences, Engineering, and Medicine, 2016, p. 153).

4. Two-way communication with key groups has been hampered "by a lack of next steps for individuals to accomplish meaningful action" (National Academies of Sciences, Engineering, and Medicine, 2016, p. 153).

5. The Campaign must disseminate communications through "health policy and business reporters, editors, and columnists at national, state, and local news outlets; and bloggers who cover issues related to the recommendations of *The Future of Nursing*" (National Academies of Sciences, Engineering, and Medicine, 2016, p. 154).

6. Training courses for spokespersons would "teach nurses how to successfully handle media interviews, lead and manage collaborative efforts with physicians and other members of the health care team, lobby for legislative changes, negotiate contracts, and resolve workplace conflicts" (National Academies of Sciences, Engineering, and Medicine, 2016, p. 154).

Study Committee's Conclusion

"For the Campaign to progress further, its communication strategy needs to expand beyond the nursing profession to other diverse stakeholders, including consumers" (National Academies of Sciences, Engineering, and Medicine, 2016, p. 155).

Study Committee's Recommendation

"The Campaign should expand the scope of its communication strategies to connect with a broader, more diverse, consumer-oriented audience and galvanize support at the grassroots level" (National Academies of Sciences, Engineering, and Medicine, 2016, p. 156).

Nurses' Vision
Do you lead change to advance health for the public?

1. Yes = 43.86% (100 respondents)

2. No = 56.14% (128 respondents)

Comments

1. "I am also an Albert Schweitzer Fellow (ASF) mentor, and I look for students who will join the fellowship to make a change for their community. People do not want to make changes, and they only want you to do so within their community culture."

2. "Communication is a barrier."

3. "I volunteer at health fair opportunities! Create areas of health within your social circle or neighborhood. As a community, we need to invest in community gardens, promote community centers, and decrease cost for health services."

4. "Barriers include cost, food desserts, lack of transportation, lack of resources. The way the food stamp program is set up, people can get frozen pizzas and sugar drinks cheaper than apples. New York took a stand on soda pop, and Vermont passed GMO standards. We need to do the same! Education and opportunity needs to start at the WIC office and in family health clinics."

5. "On a 1:1 basis with patients."

6. "Providing nurses with tools to perform more effective patient education helps to improve the well-being of the community. I also provide programs for CE (continuing education) for nurses to ensure their practice is current, which improves public health."

7. "Nurses should be prepared to redesign care delivery and payment systems by public policy master's and PhD, leadership studies, community volunteerism. Nurses need to be valued and present at the higher levels of organizational design—not just the CNO."

8. "Nurses should be prepared by understanding health promotion/illness prevention, public health as a social and financial concern, and continued patient and family education."

9. "Nurses should have paid fellowships with executives and legislators, even possibly outside of healthcare."

Do you understand the impact of payment systems on your nursing practice?

1. Yes = 52.61% (121 respondents)

2. No = 46.09% (106 respondents)

3. Other (please specify) = 1.30% (three respondents)

Comments

1. "As nurses, we still need more understanding of this and how it impacts the work we do."

2. "I understand reimbursements have impacted my charting and turned it from a communication tool among staff to a billing platform with the click checkbox charting. It is extremely demoralizing and decreases my confidence in doing my job immensely. Payment systems have improved complications from catheters or inpatient hospital-acquired pneumonia, and that's good. Requiring me to do redundant charting for the sake of billing is hamstringing my practice and significantly decreasing my direct patient care."

3. "Somewhat, but as nurses move into the community and payment models change, I will need to learn more."

Are there stakeholders outside nursing to help move the profession forward in the 2020s?

1. Yes = 44.00% (99 respondents)

2. No = 48.00% (108 respondents)

3. Other (please specify) = 8.00% (18 respondents)

Comments

1. "Consumers."

2. "Unsure." (×10)

3. "I don't know." (×6)

4. "I don't know that others outside of nursing truly have the profession's best interests at heart."

5. "All other possible collaborators who have a vested interest in the care of patients. Pharmacy, business, lab, physicians, etc."

6. "Because we are nonprofit, we have a duty to support and represent all members of the communities we serve. If we are going to educate our patients on positive change, we need to collaborate with pharmacies, physicians, food vendors, community centers, disability services . . . we need to work to empower citizens and remove barriers to care."

7. "Technology companies → healthcare is evolving; insurance companies → drive care being provided; data analysis → because of technology, we have large amounts of data, but need assistance using it."

Are you being prepared to serve in an executive or leadership position in the 2020s?

1. Yes = 33.33% (76 respondents)

2. No = 66.67% (152 respondents)

Comments

1. "Currently Assistant Nursing Director."

2. "I am a clinical professor at a nursing university."

3. "Currently in an executive nursing role."

4. "Currently in a leadership/executive position."

5. "I believe classes at the university are now looking at how to change policies and how to effect that change."

6. "Already am."

7. "I see myself teaching someone else to take over my role and effect changes."

8. "No, I will likely still be in the same role and working to make changes. Also, senior leadership is not turning over yet."

9. "I am passionate about the opportunity to work through a new delivery of care model. Those that rock the boat are normally drowned by an organization."

CHAPTER 9

Build an Infrastructure for the Collection and Analysis of Interprofessional Health Care Workforce Data (2010)

"Miss Nightingale's mastery of the art of marshalling facts to logical conclusions was recognized by her election in 1858 as a member of the Statistical Society." —E. T. Cook (Cook, 1913a, p. 387)

"A fondness for statistical method,
a belief in its almost illimitable efficacy,
was one of her marked characteristics."
—E. T. Cook (Cook, 1913a, p. 428)

NIGHTINGALE'S VISION

Florence Nightingale was dismayed by how careless military officials were in keeping statistics during her work in the Crimea. When she returned to England, she began studying hospital statistics in London. She discovered that there were no uniform hospital statistics. Each hospital had its own language to classify diseases. Numerous observations were recorded with no uniform standard. She collaborated with physicians and Dr. Farr of the Registrar-General's Office to develop standardized forms for hospital statistics based on a list of disease classes. She advocated adoption of her forms to "enable us to ascertain the relative mortality in different hospitals, as well as of different diseases and injuries at the same and at different ages, the relative frequency of different diseases and injuries among the classes which enter hospitals in different countries, and in different districts of the same countries" (Cook, 1913a, p. 430). She printed her model forms and persuaded several London hospitals to trial them. Her purpose was to build an infrastructure that "would

enable the mortality in hospitals, and also the mortality from particular diseases, injuries, and operations, to be ascertained with accuracy; and these facts, together with the duration of cases, would enable the value of particular methods of treatment and of special operations to be brought to statistical proof. The sanitary state of the hospital itself could likewise be ascertained" (Cook, 1913a, p. 430). The trial results validated the benefit of her forms for statistical analysis.

Nightingale and Dr. Farr presented these results at the International Statistical Congress. Then, she printed and distributed her forms to hospitals throughout England on request. Her plan for Uniform Hospital Statistics was a precursor of today's hospital data collection and analysis. It was not widely accepted in England because of the labor involved in collecting and collating data manually. Nightingale and her collaborators developed the initial infrastructure to collect and analyze healthcare data about hospital mortality years before it became accepted practice (Cook, 1913a).

"The National Health Care Workforce Commission, with oversight from the Government Accountability Office and the Health Resources and Services Administration, should lead a collaborative effort to improve research and the collection and analysis of data on health care workforce requirements. The Workforce Commission and the Health Resources and Services Administration should collaborate with state licensing boards, state nursing workforce centers, and the Department of Labor in this effort to ensure that the data are timely and publicly accessible" (IOM, 2011, p. 14).

The IOM Committee discovered that data was inadequate about "the numbers and types of health professionals currently employed, where they are employed, and in what roles" (IOM, 2011, p. 255). They reviewed available data on primary care physicians and nurses to project future demand and need for both types of providers. The ACA forecast increased demand for primary care practitioners when many physicians didn't specialize in primary care (IOM, 2011, p. 257). The Committee identified national underserved areas, particularly in rural communities, and determined that the supply of nurses must increase to meet health care needs. However, national and regional workforce data couldn't address these fundamental questions: "How many primary care providers does the nation require to deliver on its promise of more accessible, quality health care? What are the various proportions of physicians, nurses, physician assistants, and other providers that can be used to meet that need? What is the current educational capacity to meet the need, and how quickly can it be ramped up?" (IOM, 2011, p. 259).

After identifying gaps in data collection and analysis about the health care workforce, the Committee made the following recommendations:

1. Federal agencies (Workforce Commission and HRSA) and licensing boards in each state should "develop

and promulgate a standardized minimum data set across states and by professions that can be used to assess health care workforce needs by demographics, numbers, skill mix, and geographic distribution" (IOM, 2011, p. 15).

2. Federal agencies must "set standards for the collection of the minimum data set by state licensing boards; oversee, coordinate, and house the data; and make the data publicly accessible" (IOM, 2011, p. 15).

3. Federal agencies should strengthen the HRSA's "registered nurse sample survey by increasing the sample size, fielding the survey every other year, expanding the data collected on advanced practice registered nurses, and releasing survey results more quickly" (IOM, 2011, p. 15).

4. A monitoring system should be created based on "the minimum data set to systematically measure and project nursing workforce requirements by role, skill mix, region, and demographics" (IOM, 2011, p. 15).

5. Federal agencies (Workforce Commission and HRSA) should collaborate on "workforce research efforts with the Department of Labor, state and regional educators, employers, and state nursing workforce centers to identify regional health care workforce needs, and establish regional targets and plans for appropriately increasing the supply of health professionals" (IOM, 2011, p. 15).

6. The Government Accountability Office (GAO) should guarantee "that the Workforce Commission membership includes adequate nursing expertise" (IOM, 2011, p. 15).

How did these recommendations fare in the first five years after *The Future of Nursing* was published? The next section will explore the results and expectation for the future.

Improve Workforce Data Collection (2016)

"She was something of a pioneer in the graphic method of statistical presentation. In every branch of her inquiry she was equally thorough; consulting the best authorities, collecting the essential facts." —E. T. Cook (Cook, 1913a, p. 352)

"What we want is not so much (or at least not at present) an accumulation of facts as to teach the men who are to govern the country the use of statistical facts." —F. Nightingale (Cook, 1913b, p. 396)

NIGHTINGALE'S VISION

Nightingale knew that lack of data was not a hindrance to collection and analysis. Large volumes of statistical data were readily available, but not used. Through her interactions with political leaders, she realized that the Ministers in the Houses of Parliament were not cognizant of statistical methodology. They made decisions and enacted legislation without reference to the excellent statistics available to them. She believed it was imperative that these decision-makers know how to use statistics in their deliberations (Cook, 1913b). When Parliament stymied her efforts, she turned to the International Statistical Conference in 1860. She sent a letter asking that governments publish more abstracts of their statistical data. The letter was adopted as a resolution. Nightingale believed that the public must be aware of the importance of such information. In her words, "valuable reports, replete with facts and suggestions drawn up by committees, inspectors, directors, and prefects, remain unknown to the public. Government ought to take care to make itself acquainted with, and promote the diffusion of all good methods, to watch all endeavours, to encourage every improvement. With our habits and institutions, there is but one instrument endowed with energy and power sufficient to secure this salutary influence—that instrument is the press" (Cook, 1913a, p. 435).

After this, she turned her attention to England's colonies, especially India. Nightingale sent a survey of sanitary questions to every Indian military station and analyzed this data for its impact on the health of the military there and the Indian people. Her report illustrated that in-depth data collection and analysis could improve sanitation and health through the coordinated efforts of the India Commission, Nightingale, and officials (Cook, 1913b).

Progress toward IOM's Vision

The IOM Committee based its recommendations about developing an infrastructure for health care workforce data collection and analysis on a Workforce Commission that would coordinate with HRSA to achieve this goal. Although the ACA created the Commission and appointed commissioners (including one registered nurse) in 2010, Congress did not authorize funding and the Workforce Commission is not functioning. This has limited "progress on a single, coordinated national data infrastructure" (National Academies of Sciences, Engineering, and Medicine, 2016, p. 161), but activity has continued to improve workforce data collection and analysis.

Accomplishments

1. HRSA performed the first National Sample Survey of Nurse Practitioners in 2012, reported the results in 2014, and "made a public use data file available to researchers" (National Academies of Sciences, Engineering, and Medicine, 2016, p. 163).

2. HRSA has developed national projections of nursing supply and demand and created a web platform "that states can use to generate supply and demand models by entering their state-based data and other assumptions about attrition from or entrance into the profession" (National Academies of Sciences, Engineering, and Medicine, 2016, p. 163).

3. Current federal workforce data collection instruments have been expanded to include APRNs (National Academies of Sciences, Engineering, and Medicine, 2016, p. 164).

4. There has been agreement on the Minimum Data Set's data elements (National Academy of Sciences, Engineering, and Medicine, 2016, p. 164).

5. There are "34 State Nursing Workforce Centers; 30 collect supply data, 20 demand data, and 31 education data" (National Academies of Sciences, Engineering, and Medicine, 2016, p. 164).

6. The Campaign has seen progress in "the number of recommended nursing workforce data items collected by states" (National Academies of Sciences, Engineering, and Medicine, 2016, p. 165).

Challenges

1. HRSA is no longer conducting a survey of registered nurses (National Academies of Sciences, Engineering, and Medicine, 2016, p. 163).

2. State Nursing Workforce Centers are not available in 16 states (National Academies of Sciences, Engineering, and Medicine, 2016, p. 164).

3. There is no "overall infrastructure for the collection and analysis of data on the nursing or interprofessional health workforce" (National Academies of Sciences, Engineering, and Medicine, 2016, p. 167).

4. Existing health workforce data sources are not uniform and include gaps, such as data collected about physicians' practices that does not include information about NPs employed in these practices (National Academies of Sciences, Engineering, and Medicine, 2016, p. 167).

5. There is "lag time in the collection and reporting of data" (National Academies of Sciences, Engineering, and Medicine, 2016, p. 166).

6. Data on the services NPs provide and their care settings is not comprehensive because many NPs with collaborative agreements or employed by hospitals do not use their own National Provider Identifier (NPI) to bill for services (National Academies of Sciences, Engineering, and Medicine, 2016, p. 166).

Study Committee's Conclusion

"Numerous health professional organizations have urged funding of the National Health Care Workforce Commission and have been active in bolstering workforce data collection with their own professions. These efforts suggest that common ground and interprofessional collaboration may be achieved to advance this recommendation of *The Future of Nursing*" (National Academies of Sciences, Engineering, and Medicine, 2016, p. 171).

Study Committee's Recommendation

"The Campaign should promote collaboration among organizations that collect workforce-related data. Given the absence of the National Health Care Workforce Commission, the Campaign can use its strong brand and partnerships to help improve the collection of data on the nursing workforce" (National Academies of Sciences, Engineering, and Medicine, 2016, p. 172).

Nurses' Vision

Are you involved in data collection and/or analysis related to nursing professional practice?

1. Yes = 39.30% (90 respondents)

2. No = 60.70% (139 respondents)

Comments

1. "Unsure."

2. "Need a mobile application that individuals could update in addition to organizations—degree statistics, length of employment, certifications held."

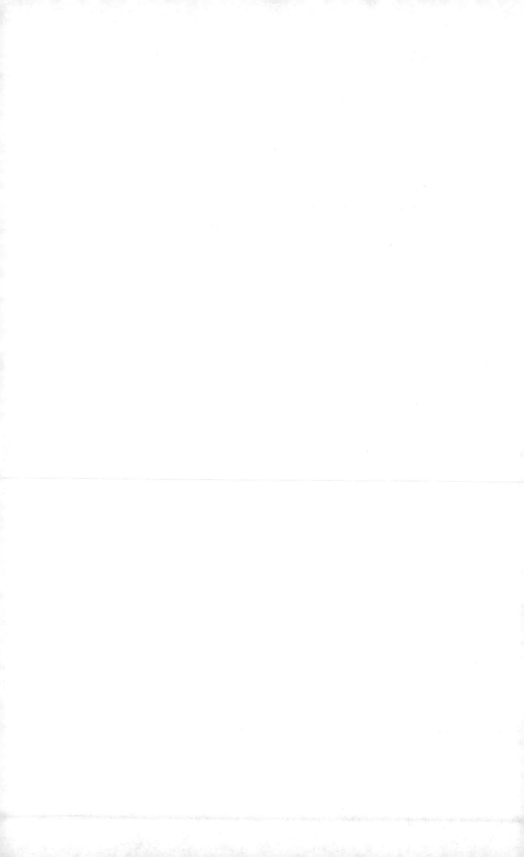

Where Do We Go from Here?

Health care and nursing continue to evolve as we approach the third decade of the twenty-first century. The Patient Protection and Affordable Care Act still exists but cannot continue unchanged. Currently, discussion is underway about repeal and replacement of the ACA and health-care reform in the future. Despite its limitations, the ACA provided opportunities for nurses to practice to the extent of their license in multiple settings. Its passage in 2010 also fueled the Institute of Medicine (IOM) recommendations in *The Future of Nursing*. These recommendations were refined by the Study Committee of 2015, and the Future of Nursing Campaign for Action continues to implement them via the Center to Champion Nursing in America (CCNA), which collaborates with State Action Coalitions to meet its goals (National Academies of Sciences, Engineering, and Medicine, 2016, p. 2).

Nursing experiences both triumphs and challenges that must be addressed for the profession to advance in the 2020s. For the 15th year in a row, nurses are the most trusted profession as well as the largest (>3.6 million) group of healthcare providers (ANA, 2017). Yet they were excluded from an initial healthcare reform meeting with healthcare executives and the administration (Thew, 2017). Many of the issues—access to care, transitional care, managing chronic illnesses, cost containment, ambulatory care, health promotion, preventive services—are linked to availability of nurses who are educationally prepared to coordinate and provide care in community as well as acute care settings. The availability of such registered nurses depends on the success of the IOM recommendations related to the following:

1. Removing scope-of-practice barriers (IOM, 2011)

2. Opportunities to lead and diffuse collaborative improvement efforts (IOM, 2011)

3. Presence of nurse residency and nurse fellowship programs (IOM, 2011)

4. Increasing the number of nurses with baccalaureate and higher degrees (MSNs, DNPs, PhDs) (IOM, 2011)

5. Engagement of nurses in lifelong learning (IOM, 2011)

6. Developing nurses to lead change to advance health (IOM, 2011)

7. Building an infrastructure to collect and analyze inter-professional health care workforce data (IOM, 2011)

For these initiatives to succeed, nurses at all levels must hone their leadership and interprofessional collaboration skills using the IOM recommendations and the Study Committee's identified focus areas (Academies of Sciences, Engineering, and Medicine, 2016). The nurses who participated in the survey for this book were asked one final, very important question: What change(s) would you recommend to advance nursing in the 2020s?

Readers will agree with some of their responses and disagree with others. What is important is that they have honestly shared their predictions and hopes for nursing's future. These nurses will lead the profession into the 2020s and beyond. Their voice needs to be heard.

What change(s) would you recommend to advance nursing in the 2020s?

1. Promotion of lifelong learning/education = 58.85% (133 respondents)

2. Leadership development at all levels = 64.16% (145 respondents)

3. Better data collection/utilization related to nursing professional practice = 41.15% (93 respondents)

4. Better interprofessional collaboration = 61.50% (139 respondents)

5. Greater involvement in care delivery redesign = 72.57% (164 respondents)

Comments

1. "With research utilizing nanoparticles—specialized nursing care is going to exist in the nonhospital setting. Home and nursing home advanced practice nurses would alleviate readmission rates. The ability to coach and educate on a personal level would help. As healthcare workers, we need to advocate for better school lunches and preventative actions. Current healthcare is reactive—the new model will have proactive measures."

2. "Use of technology could change the way we determine competence."

3. "I would hope we can use telehealth as nurses to better reach all types of people. More people seem to know about technology even though our baby boomers like more face-to-face than the millennials."

4. "Something that would help encourage nurses to advance is some kind of motivation. Right now, we are asked to get our BSN only because of the IOM, but there is no pay raise involved, no acknowledgement, nothing. Just debt. Motivation would help, but until then, the % of nurses getting their BSN is not as great as it could be."

5. "More integrated nursing care options."

6. "More focus on prevention/public health in nursing education would be amazing. From my experience, this area is largely underrepresented. Prevention saves lives, enhances quality of life, and is cost effective. Bedside nursing is incredibly important too, but my hope is that the nursing profession will take a progressive perspective and start placing more value on the power of prevention."

7. "More competent training for our new nurses coming in to all settings as well as for experienced nurses spreading their wings with new challenges in all settings, including not just inpatient care."

8. "Funding."

9. "Better staffing ratios for bedside nursing in hospital settings and more support from management."

10. "Mandatory safe nurse/patient ratios." (×2)

11. "Have more respect for bedside nursing and share with others the importance of bedside nursing. I feel nurses are pressured to move up the ladder and get away from bedside nursing."

12. "I feel like I get no leadership training at all."

13. "Develop methods to establish nursing as a profession vs. a skill set. Increase respect within the medical community for nursing, especially bedside nursing."

14. "More staff at bedside, so we can do these things. Address burnout to keep the nurses we have, or 2020 won't even matter."

15. "Nurse leadership in the implementation of evidence-based nursing practice."

16. "Funds for further education and increase in salary for recognition."

17. "Nursing practice OUTSIDE of traditional health care facilities (e.g., community, FQHC, public and private schools, charter schools, etc.)."

Florence Nightingale would be 200 years old in 2020, which is also a pivotal year for the IOM recommendations. Nightingale's vision has guided nursing practice to the present day. Today's nurses will advance the profession to a new chapter in 2020 and beyond.

APPENDIX A

Survey Questions

Nightingale's Vision & the IOM (Institute of Medicine) Recommendations

Nursing in the 2020s—Feedback from RNs ages 25–45

Nightingale's vision for the profession reflects the 2010 Institute of Medicine (IOM) recommendations for nursing and the 2015 Assessment Report in education, nursing leadership, interprofessional collaboration, data collection/utilization, lifelong learning, and involvement in care delivery redesign. This survey is an opportunity for nurses 25–45 to determine nursing's future.

1. What is your level of knowledge about the IOM (Institute of Medicine) recommendations for nursing?

( ) Know nothing about them

( ) Have skimmed the recommendations—minimal knowledge level

( ) Have read and understand the recommendations—competent knowledge level

( ) Involved in the implementation of the recommendations—expert knowledge level

2. Are you able to practice to the limits of your license?

( ) Yes

( ) No

Other (please specify)

[   ]

3. Do you lead interprofessional (involving other professions and nursing) collaborative improvement projects?

( ) Yes

( ) No

Other (please specify)

[   ]

4. Does your healthcare setting have a transition-to-practice residency for new RNs?

( ) Yes

( ) No

Other (please specify)

[   ]

5. Does your healthcare setting have a fellowship program for advanced practice nurses?

- ◯ Yes
- ◯ No

Other (please specify)

[   ]

6. Is your healthcare setting on track to meet the IOM recommendation of 80% BSNs by 2020?

- ◯ Yes
- ◯ No

Other (please specify)

[   ]

7. Another recommendation is to double the number of nurses with doctorates by 2020. Do you or other RNs in your healthcare setting have a doctoral degree (PhD, DNP)?

- ◯ Yes
- ◯ No

Other (please specify)

[   ]

8. Does your healthcare setting support lifelong learning as a priority for nurses?

- ◯ Yes
- ◯ No

Other (please specify)

[   ]

9. Do you lead change to advance health for the public?

- ◯ Yes
- ◯ No

Other (please specify)

[   ]

10. Does your healthcare setting make diversity a priority in workforce hiring and retention?

○ Yes

○ No

Other (please specify)

[ ]

11. Are you involved in data collection and/or analysis related to nursing professional practice?

○ Yes

○ No

Other (please specify)

[ ]

12. Are there stakeholders outside nursing to help move the profession forward in the 2020s?

○ Yes

○ No

○ Other (please specify)

[ ]

13. Are you being prepared to serve in an executive or leadership position in the 2020s?

○ Yes

○ No

Other (please specify)

[ ]

14. Do you understand the impact of payment systems on your nursing practice?

○ Yes

○ No

○ Other (please specify)

[ ]

15. What change(s) would you recommend to advance nursing in the 2020s?

☐ promotion of lifelong learning/education

☐ leadership development at all levels

☐ better data collection/utilization related to nursing professional practice

☐ better interprofessional collaboration

☐ greater involvement in care delivery redesign

Other (please specify)

[   ]

APPENDIX B

Survey Data

Q1 What is your level of knowledge about the IOM (Institute of Medicine) recommendations for nursing?

Answered: 232   Skipped: -1

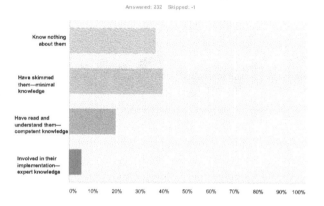

Answer Choices	Responses	
Know nothing about them	**36.21%**	84
Have skimmed the recommendations—minimal knowledge level	**39.22%**	91
Have read and understand the recommendations—competent knowledge level	**19.40%**	45
Involved in the implementation of the recommendations—expert knowledge level	**5.17%**	12
Total		**232**

Q2 Are you able to practice to the limits of your license?

Answered: 230   Skipped: 1

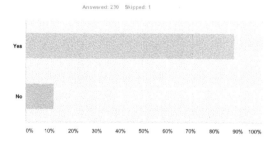

Answer Choices	Responses	
Yes	**88.26%**	203
No	**11.74%**	27
Total		**230**

Q3 Do you lead interprofessional (involving other professions and nursing) collaborative improvement projects?

Answered: 231   Skipped: 0

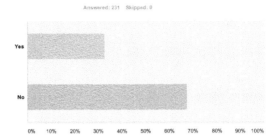

Answer Choices	Responses	
Yes	32.47%	75
No	67.53%	156
Total		231

Q4 Does your healthcare setting have a transition-to-practice residency for new RNs?

Answered: 225   Skipped: 5

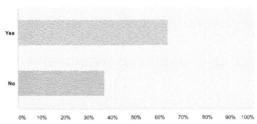

Answer Choices	Responses	
Yes	63.56%	143
No	36.44%	82
Total		225

Q5 Does your healthcare setting have a fellowship program for advanced practice nurses?

Answered: 210   Skipped: 21

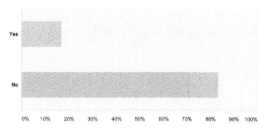

Answer Choices	Responses	
Yes	16.67%	35
No	83.33%	175
Total		210

Q6 Is your heathcare setting on track to meet the IOM recommendation of 80% BSNs by 2020?

Answered: 203   Skipped: 28

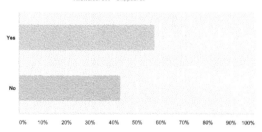

Answer Choices	Responses	
Yes	57.14%	116
No	42.86%	87
Total		203

Q7 Another recommendation is to double the number of nurses with doctorates by 2020. Do you or other RNs in your healthcare setting have a doctoral degree (PhD, DNP)?

Answered: 225   Skipped: 6

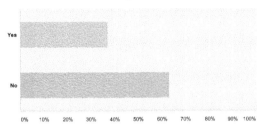

Answer Choices	Responses	
Yes	36.89%	83
No	63.11%	142
Total		225

Q8 Does your healthcare setting support lifelong learning as a priority for nurses?

Answered: 229   Skipped: 2

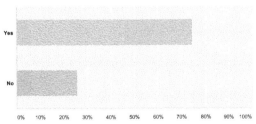

Answer Choices	Responses	
Yes	74.24%	170
No	25.76%	59
Total		229

Q9 Do you lead change to advance health for the public?

Answered: 228   Skipped: 3

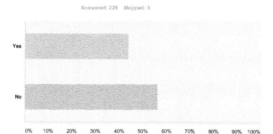

Answer Choices	Responses	
Yes	43.86%	100
No	56.14%	128
Total		228

Q10 Does your healthcare setting make diversity a priority in workforce hiring and retention?

Answered: 223   Skipped: 8

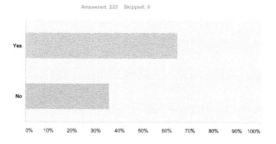

Answer Choices	Responses	
Yes	64.57%	144
No	35.43%	79
Total		223

Q11 Are you involved in data collection and/or analysis related to nursing professional practice?

Answered: 229 Skipped: 2

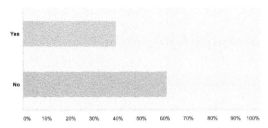

Answer Choices	Responses	
Yes	39.30%	90
No	60.70%	139
Total		229

Q12 Are there stakeholders outside nursing to help move the profession forward in the 2020s?

Answered: 225 Skipped: 6

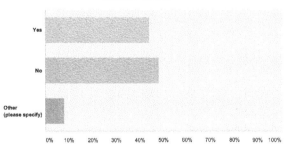

Answer Choices	Responses	
Yes	44.00%	99
No	48.00%	108
Other (please specify)	8.00%	18
Total		225

Q13 Are you being prepared to serve in an executive or leadership position in the 2020s?

Answered: 228   Skipped: 3

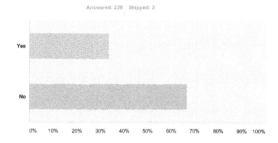

Answer Choices	Responses	
Yes	33.33%	76
No	66.67%	152
Total		228

Q14 Do you understand the impact of payment systems on your nursing practice?

Answered: 230   Skipped: 1

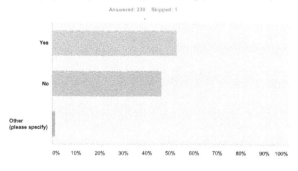

Answer Choices	Responses	
Yes	52.61%	121
No	46.09%	106
Other (please specify)	1.30%	3
Total		230

Q15 What change(s) would you recommend to advance nursing in the 2020s?

Answered: 226   Skipped: 5

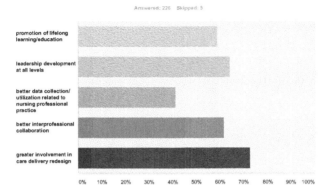

Answer Choices	Responses	
promotion of lifelong learning/education	58.85%	133
leadership development at all levels	64.16%	145
better data collection/utilization related to nursing professional practice	41.15%	93
better interprofessional collaboration	61.50%	139
greater involvement in care delivery redesign	72.57%	164
Total Respondents: 226		

References

American Nurses Association. (2017). *About ANA*. Retrieved March 2017, from American Nurses Association: http://www .nursingworld.org/

Center to Champion Nursing. (2011). *Increasing Diversity in Nursing*. Retrieved January 3, 2017, from Campaign for Action: http:// Campaignforaction.org

Cook, E. T. (1913a). *The Life of Florence Nightingale* (Vol. 1). London: Macmillan and Co., Ltd.

Cook, E. T. (1913b). *The Life of Florence Nightingale* (Vol. 2). London: Macmillan and Co., Ltd.

Department of Veterans Affairs. (2016, December 14). *Rules and Regulations*. Retrieved January 17, 2017, from Federal Register: gpo.gov

Institute of Medicine. (2011). *The Future of Nursing: Leading Change, Advancing Health*. Washington, DC: National Academies Press.

IOM (Institute of Medicine). (2011). *A Summary of the February 2010 Forum on the Future of Nursing: Education*. Washington, DC: The National Academies Press.

Judd, D., Sitzman, K., & Davis, G. (2010). *A History of American Nursing: Trends and Eras*. Sudbury, MA: Jones and Bartlett Publishers.

National Academies of Sciences, Engineering, and Medicine. (2016). *Assessing Progress on the Institute of Medicine Report: The Future of Nursing*. Washington, DC: The National Academies Press.

Nightingale, F. (2012). *Florence Nightingale to Her Nurses (Originally published in 1914)*. Forgotten Books. Retrieved from www.forgottenbooks.org

Thew, J. (2017, February 1). *Nurses Missing from Healthcare Reform Talks*. Retrieved February 2, 2017, from Health Leaders Media: www.healthleadersmedia.com

We're Building a Healthier America Through Nursing. (2010). Retrieved January 6, 2017, from Campaign for Action: http:// campaignforaction.org/

Index

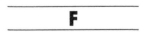

O

P